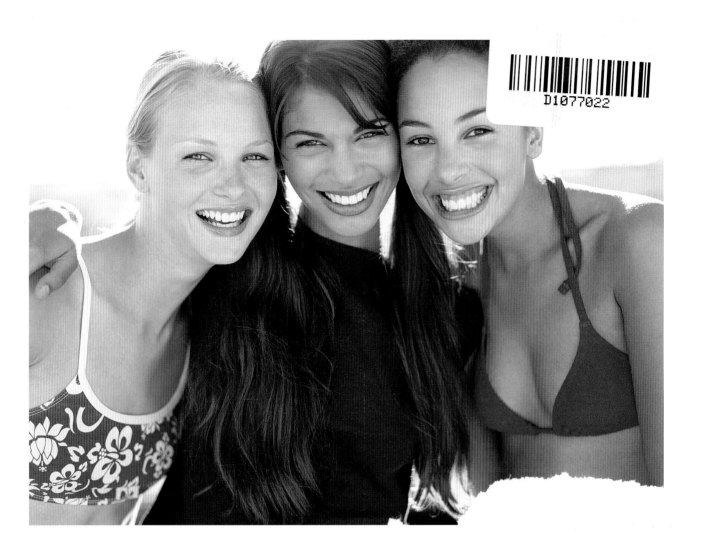

GO FOR IT!

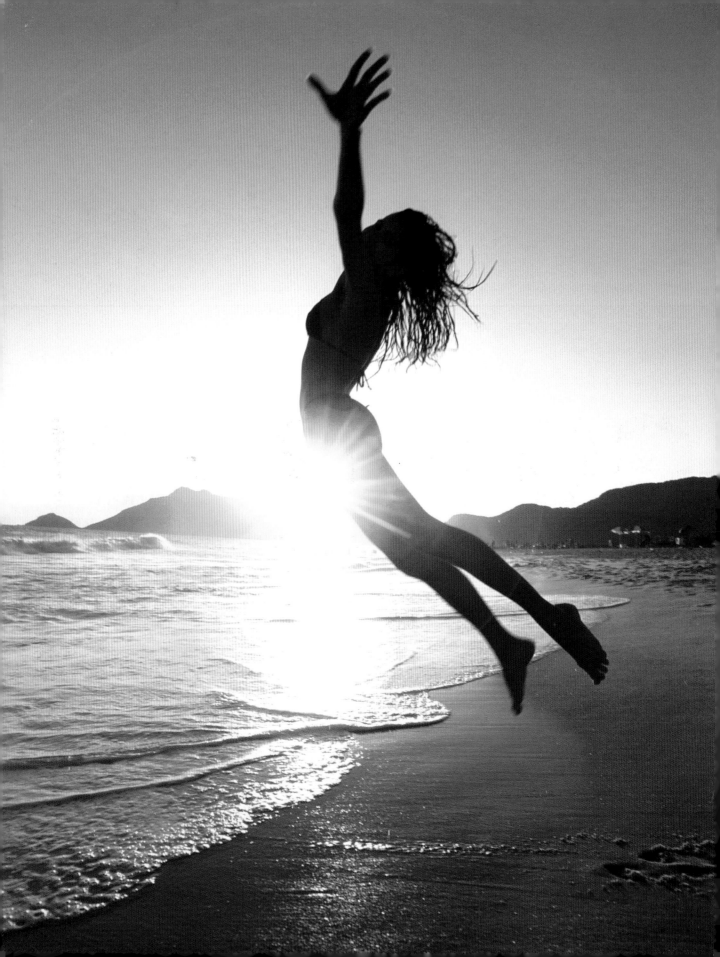

dawna walter

GO FOR IT!

sort your life! achieve your dreams! have fun!

quadrille

Editorial Director: Jane O'Shea
Creative Director: Helen Lewis
Project Editor: Lisa Pendreigh
Designer: Jim Smith
Illustrator: Coralie Bickford-Smith
Picture Researcher: Nadine Bazar and Jim Smith
Production Controller: Tracy Hart

First published in 2003 by
Quadrille Publishing Ltd
Alhambra House
27–31 Charing Cross Road
London WC2H 0LS

Cataloguing-in-Publication Data: a catalogue record for this
book is available from the British Library.

ISBN 1 844000 13 3

Printed and bound by by C & C Offset in China.

contents

introduction

Go For It! is a very personal book that embodies a philosophy I have practiced ever since I can remember. Six words come to mind when I think of 'going for it', or giving what you desire your best efforts: imagination, expectation, stimulation, creation, appreciation and observation. If you can imagine your heart's desire and believe that you can have it, by focussing your energy on what you want and ignoring all of the negatives, you will get it.

Look back at any achievement in your life and remember the steps you took to get there. I bet each of us can remember really wanting to accomplish a goal and working hard to achieve it. There may have been someone in your life at that time that believed in you and urged you on. Or maybe you just had to prove to yourself that you could do it. Either way, the feeling of being excited by something is unbeatable.

Throughout my life I have had many big dreams that I realised through my sheer belief that they were attainable. With this attitude, I rarely saw obstacles but looked for ways to accomplish my goals. I was a woman on a mission, creating my vision and having fun in the process. I was not always successful, but it never stopped me from beginning something else with the greatest enthusiasm. It is always the journey that makes life interesting.

I have also had times in my life with no clear vision of what I wanted. After graduating from university, I spent a year unable to focus my attention on anything. Thinking about too many things at one time leads to confusion.

This confusion can lead to loss of energy, motivation and even physical illness. One day I realised that I wanted to feel better and have clearer vision, and rather than worry about what I was going to do for the rest of my life, I was able to look at short-term wishes rather than long-term dreams. By accomplishing small things, you start

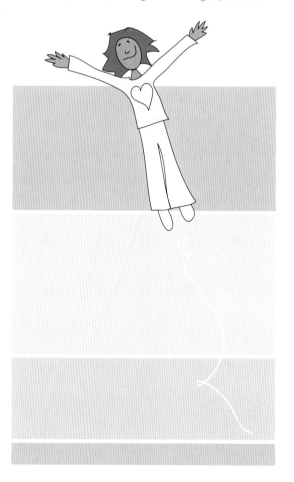

feeling better about yourself and are able to achieve more by simply believing that you can.

Anyone can easily shift from confusion to clarity by focussing on one thing at a time. As you face each situation in the day, choose to feel good and see the positive aspects. Decide what you want to achieve and do not worry about what others do. Going for it means having a dream or a vision of what you want, even if it is what you want for just one day, and enthusiastically going about getting it.

When we do things with passion, they are definitely more fun and not surprisingly, seem to take little effort. Abraham Lincoln said, 'Laughter is the joyous, beautiful, universal evergreen of life.' Finding something to laugh about or having fun in each situation makes an enormous difference to how you feel. When you are feeling good, you are in harmony with what you desire, which is to get the most out of each situation.

We feel best when our physical and emotional beings are in harmony. We feel balanced when we have thoughts and ideas that we are able to create into reality. When we have an idea that we are excited about, we begin to use our imaginations to look at all the ways of getting it done. The more excited we become about the idea, the more we talk about it and can envision it happening. Everything always seems to fall into place to help when you are enthused about what you are doing.

By getting in a great frame of mind before beginning anything and thinking about what you want from the situation, you will see only that which you want to see. Being positive feels much better than being negative. When we feel good, we have just the right amount of energy. We have ideas and dreams and act on them. We are able to communicate well with those around us and know how to look after ourselves. We feel happy.

Sometimes there may be areas of our life in which we do not feel happy or balanced. When we worry, feel angry or unwell physically, our energy is concentrated on the negative aspect of the situation. It is often difficult, especially if there is physical pain, to concentrate on anything else. However, this way of thinking makes the situation worse. It often causes a lack of energy that makes it difficult to focus on anything.

Without realising it, we are often thinking in a negative way about some aspects of our lives – work, family life in the home, relationships, health or money. We all know that when we worry about something we generally do not feel very good. We may be unable to sleep or eat properly or lack the energy to get through a busy day. These are all signs that how we are thinking is not harmonious with what we desire. Just by paying attention to whatever you are thinking about when you are feeling ill at ease, you can understand those thoughts that are not harmonious with your real desires.

We also spend a lot of time thinking about what we 'need', such as a companion, a better job, more money or anything that we feel a lack of in our life. This feeling of need does not make you feel good physically or emotionally, therefore, it is not in harmony with your desires. Need looks at what you do not have. When you focus on what you lack, you are not creating what you want. Shifting your thoughts towards what you want will help to create that experience.

In all of my professional experiences looking at people's material possessions and helping them on their path of well-being, I have found that when people lose their enthusiasm in life, it is reflected in everything around them. They stop paying attention and problems start building up. This can amount to clutter in their house, or them simply thinking about too many things at once and not being able to accomplish any one project. All of the methods used in this book have worked for those that have come to me seeking solutions. As soon as you start searching for the answers rather than dwelling on the problems, you will find what you want.

Dawna Walter, February 2003

time for **change**

"Whatever you do or dream you can do – begin it.
Boldness has genius and power and magic in it."

Johann Goethe

The greatest motivation to change your circumstances often results from lacking something in your life. You run out of time or space, you do not have an ideal body or relationship, you feel unappreciated in your job, you lack energy or enthusiasm.

In actuality, everything you are living in the present moment is a direct result of your past beliefs and thoughts. From the time you were little, you have been shaped by others' opinions of your abilities. If from childhood your closest relatives and friends have inspired and encouraged you to believe that you can achieve all that you desire, in all odds you will have a positive, go-getting attitude. You will have learnt to focus your attention on the present as a stepping-stone for where you would like to be in the future, and can integrate this confidence or positive thinking into most aspects of your life. If, however, your childhood was filled with people pointing out all of your faults and lesser abilities, you may believe that you are not worthy of those things that you truly desire. As is often the case, the more negative belief patterns that you hold, the less likely you are to achieve your dreams, but even worse, to dare to dream them.

Your thoughts and feelings are indications of how well you are doing in achieving the things you desire. When you feel good physically, mentally and emotionally, this is a clear indication that you are in harmony with your innermost desires. Often you notice that when all is well in a given area of life, you go from strength to strength. Positive thoughts seem to attract more positive thoughts and, coincidentally, you seem to see and hear more information that reinforce your thoughts, helping you on your way. This is your inner wisdom, or inner guidance system, saying 'well done'.

When you feel bad physically, mentally or emotionally, what you are thinking about in that moment is at the root of the problem, as these thoughts or feelings are not in harmony with your desires. Most likely you will find that you spend your time looking at the problems rather than for solutions. We all have experienced the kind of day that goes from bad to worse, or got into a downward spiral in some area of our lives. Upon close inspection you will find that you expected the worse to happen and it did. Simply put, you must switch the focus from looking at what you do not want, to that which you do want.

Anyone who wishes to get rid of old beliefs can do so, even those who have deeply ingrained negative beliefs and feelings from childhood. Simply by learning to pay attention to how you feel in each aspect of your day, you can begin to learn what makes you feel good. The goal is to find something in each situation that makes you feel good – then anything can be achieved.

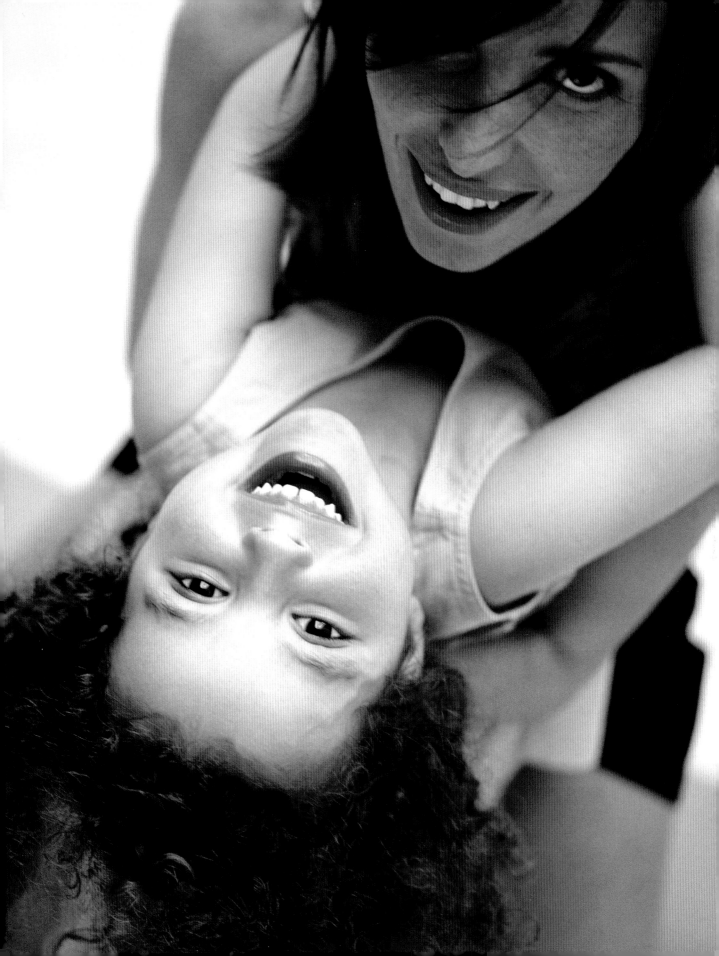

tune into your feelings

Feelings are experienced on many different levels – mental, physical, emotional and spiritual. When you are happy in all you do, these feelings are integrated and balanced. Happiness is a sign that what you are thinking and feeling in that moment is in harmony with your desires. If you find happiness in your current work, it is an indication that you are doing the job that you are meant to do to achieve your long-term goals. If you are happy listening to music, it may elevate your imagination and bring you to a higher place spiritually. If you are happy developing your body, you have learned to appreciate being physical. If you are happy in your personal relationships, you have learned to look at things in a loving way.

When you feel good on the physical level, you are comfortable with your body and are in good health. You have energy for activities but are able to relax when you need to rest. You understand the causal relationship between how you feel and the food you put into your body. Feeling good mentally means you are able to think clearly about things. You can accomplish many tasks in a day by focusing your attention, and can see a project through to completion. You think about what you want and are receptive to new ideas, which may help you to get it. You listen to your intuition, or inner guidance.

Being happy feels wonderful; everything else just does not compare. This contrast can provide the impetus to want to feel better, as looking and feeling physically bad is an indication that your body is out of balance and change is required. When you feel bad on the bodily level, either with your appearance or with a physical condition that seems ever present, you give a lot of your attention to these feelings.

When you have dis-ease, it may mean that a part of your being is ill at ease with all that you are thinking about. As we have all experienced when we feel physically ill, it is very difficult to take your attention away from the actual pain. The more you focus on the pain, however, the worse it becomes and it is not until you sleep that you are able to forget your discomfort and allow your body to heal.

Some conditions, such as eating disorders, digestive problems, allergies, skin irritations or Chronic Fatigue Syndrome, or ME, can be your body's response to excessive worry or negative thinking. After consultation with a doctor, you may find that stress or emotional issues, rather than physical problems with your body, cause these conditions. It is often difficult to get over them as they seem to take over your life, occupying your thoughts most of the time. This is a giant wake-up call from your inner guidance telling you that what you are thinking about is not harmonious with your innermost desires.

By thinking about these conditions negatively, they remain the same or even worsen. It is difficult to muster energy when you are feeling unwell, but the more static you become, the less energy you have. Enthusiasm and joy is often lost, leading to more negative thoughts. You can then get angry and frustrated, adding more negative emotion, until it becomes difficult to find a way forward.

In the course of a hectic life, we all neglect our bodies by either not eating properly or over-indulging.

Usually the side effects of this lifestyle, such as a hangover, cause you to take notice and change your habits. You pay attention to your inner guidance system. Sometimes the symptoms can be quite easy to fix, as with some headaches that are a result of not taking the time to eat properly and drink water throughout the day. Again, the body is signalling you that you must become more aware of how food nourishes and provides the physical stamina to propel you forward. As soon as you eat and drink water, the headache goes away.

Other symptoms are more debilitating, such as Chronic Fatigue Syndrome, or ME, resulting in a lack of energy that makes the gentlest activity exhausting. These illnesses can often occur several years after a traumatic event or turning point in life. It often gives you the feeling of being disconnected from the earth and unfocused. It takes a conscious effort to stop thinking about how you do feel and want to feel better.

Many of us have a difficult relationship with food, but this is not surprising if we consider popular attitudes to eating. People who are heavier than they would like may fear that each bite is going to make them fatter, whereas people who have many food intolerances may worry that everything they eat will give them a reaction. More often than not, they fulfil their expectations.

The more we talk about our dis-satisfaction, the more we add to it emotions such as anger, hatred, jealousy, or sorrow, which makes us feel more deeply, intensifies negative feelings and attracts more of the same into our lives. Emotions come from the subconscious level and many of the emotions we experience throughout our lives have been learned over time. Positive emotions, such as love, joy and appreciation, make our dreams come to us more quickly as when we experience these emotions we are looking at things that please us. The more we can find ways in each thing we do to bring love, joy and appreciation, the more we will enjoy the process of growing and having new dreams.

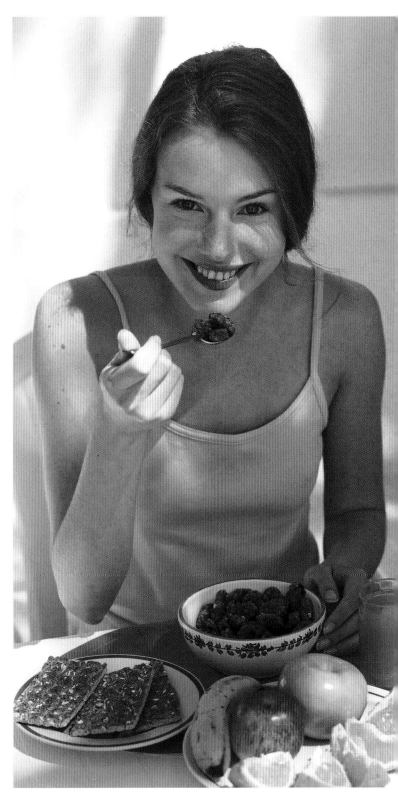

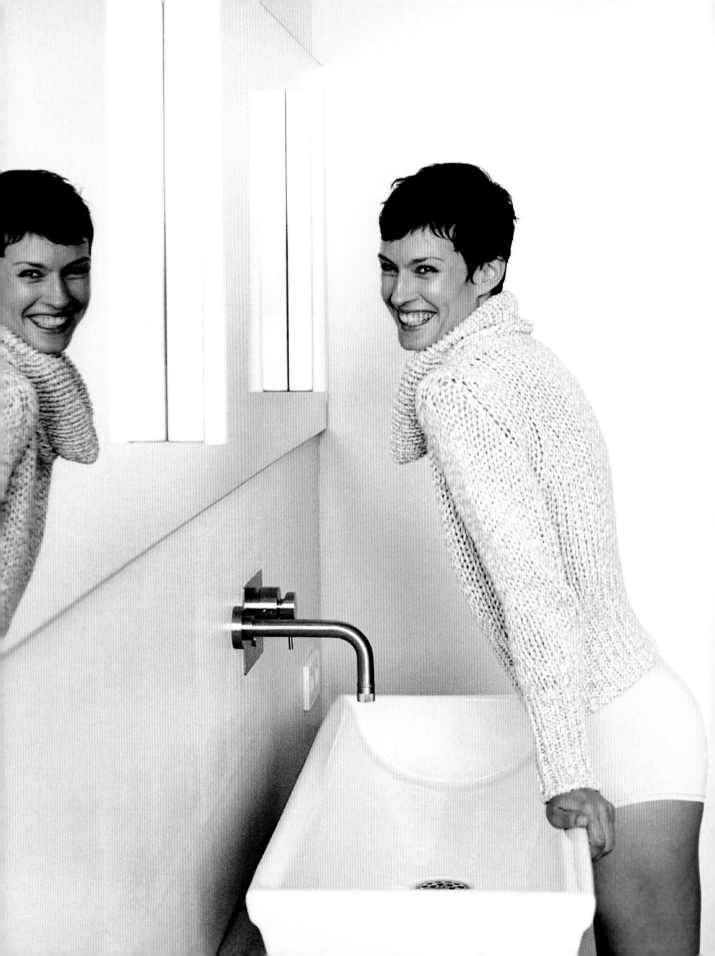

choose to feel better

If your physical state is preventing you achieving your dreams, it is important to consciously choose to feel better each day. Your thoughts are powerful attractors of how you feel, so by changing what you think about when you experience physical discomfort, you can begin to pave the way towards feeling better each day.

Your inner guidance makes it easy to know when you are on the right path to achieving your innermost desires. Whenever you are on track, you are rewarded by feeling good in appearance, condition and energy levels. The more joyous and appreciative you are of the process, the better you feel. As this feeling spreads to all that you encounter, you find that you easily accomplish your goals.

Whenever you are feeling bad, your guidance is telling you that, in that moment, you are not moving forward with what you really want. Your thoughts or emotions are holding you back. In recognising the physical symptoms of dis-ease, you can change how you are thinking at the time of experiencing discomfort. In most circumstances, the worry or attention paid to feelings perpetuates them.

When you change your reaction to a situation, you change how your body responds forever. If, for example, you experience an upset stomach every time you attend a meeting, by changing your reaction just once, your expectations have changed and the cycle has been broken. In every situation you enter, you have a choice: to dwell on physical discomfort or to imagine feeling well. By choosing to feel better, you begin to understand that you have

the power to focus your attention on the things that you want – a healthier, happier life rather than living an experience of physical and emotional pain.

When you are thinking positive thoughts, your body reflects this. When you are happy, you laugh or smile, your body is relaxed and you are open and receptive. When you have too much stimulation, you become confused. As you think about things, you activate your imagination and, through your senses, access more information about what you are thinking about.

We are all guilty at one time in our life of thinking about too many things at one time, resulting in getting very little done. For each thing that you think about, you summon information regarding this thought. When you have many thoughts at the same time, you constantly have information coming at you. You end up thinking so much that you cannot take action. When you live 'inside your head', you do not feel a connection to what is going on around you, leaving you unbalanced and ungrounded.

Just as your thoughts play an important role in how you feel and what you get, your current ways of thinking in situations that make you feel bad, can hold you back in the areas you are ready to change.

We are all capable of learning to focus our thoughts on one thing at a time. Each and every one of us has a choice in how we think in any situation. By learning to focus your mind on one thing at a time and by choosing to feel good in every situation, there is nothing that cannot be achieved.

understand your emotions

Emotions are learned responses to situations you have experienced throughout your life, many of which have been carried over from childhood. Emotions associated with past experiences may have provided you with the contrast needed to form new emotional responses to similar circumstances.

Your emotions intensify how you feel. There are two types of emotions. Positive emotions, such as love, joy, reverence or gratitude, feel good physically, especially in the heart area. You feel a general sense of well-being; there may also be spontaneous tears of joy. In all cases, these physical responses are an indication that what you are doing or thinking about in that moment is really pleasing you.

Negative emotions also have an immediate physical effect on the body. Anger, hatred, jealousy or sorrow cause tension in the heart area, sometimes a sharp pain or elevated blood pressure. The physical discomfort of such emotions is a signal from your inner self that what you are doing or thinking about in that negative thought is not in your higher interest.

Emotions propel your thoughts more quickly, whether they are positive or negative. As you project your thoughts and emotions onto others, you are likely to receive the same emotions back. If you are feeling relaxed and joyous, you are probably surrounded by others who are sharing your mood. You attract more joy into your life by attracting people and situations that reflect and amplify your mood.

It is often the case that, in situations where you experience strong negative emotions, things can get out of control. Because emotions come from your subconscious mind, you act rather than think. The longer you hold on to the emotion, the stronger it becomes as it attracts more negative energy. When you focus on anger, hatred, jealousy or sorrow, you are choosing to see only those things in the situation. By understanding how this affects what you experience, however, you can learn to take your focus away from the things that anger you.

Belief systems are formed through experience. As you experience things in the same way over and over again, you come to expect it to always happen so. A simple example of such expectation is turning on a tap: you expect the water to flow. This often happens when searching for a job but not finding the right one. The experience of rejection soon makes you lose your enthusiasm. You stop looking because you anticipate what will happen rather than being in the moment and letting things happen naturally.

If you have stopped looking forward to new experiences, it may be an indication that you are so stuck in the past you can no longer experience what is happening in the moment. Your expectations prevent you from feeling excited, hopeful and looking forward to the positive things that can occur. You need to learn to have a bit more fun and look forward to the journey rather than the end result.

When you pay attention to the journey, you become aware of all the helpful signs along the way. As you become open and receptive to believing that you are in control of your own destiny rather than it happening by chance, you are able to learn new ways of looking at old situations.

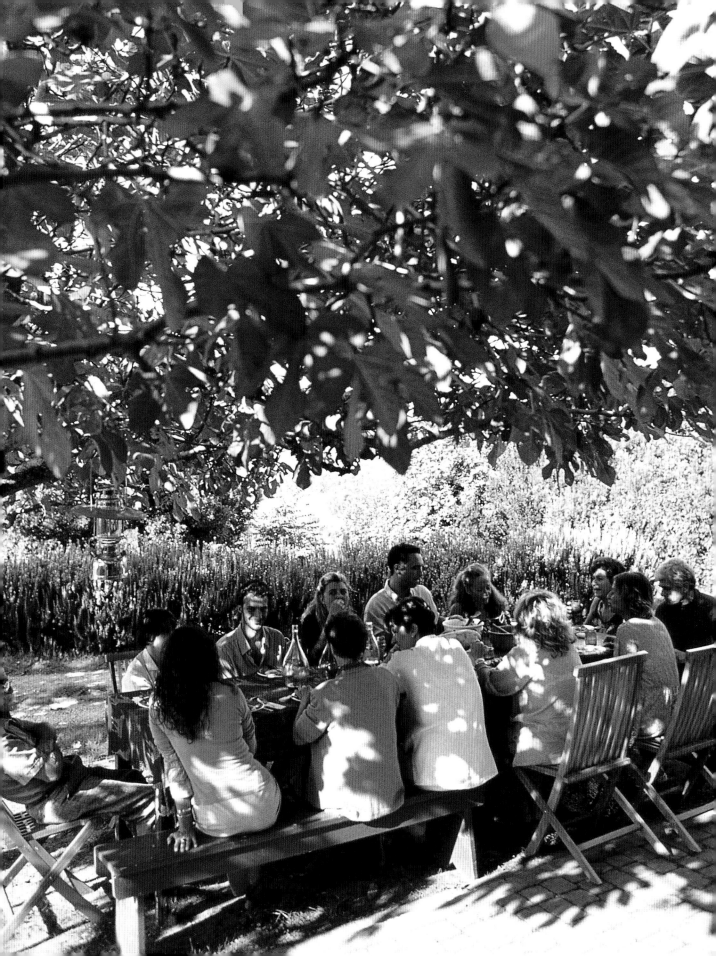

wise up

Observations of natural occurrences have been passed down through the centuries via religious doctrines, philosophies and proverbs. One such 'universal truth' is the wisdom that similar things are attracted to each other; this is reflected in the saying 'Birds of a feather flock together.' Another such expression is 'Be careful what you wish for, as you may get it.' This adage reflects a similar philosophy in that your thoughts attract the subject of your thoughts or, in other words, like attracts like.

Thought as the attractor of experience is the basis upon which the power of positive thinking is formulated. You can choose how you view each situation you encounter. Personalities are commonly categorised through a test in which a vessel is filled to the midway point with liquid. The subject is asked how they view the glass. Those who view the glass as half full tend to be more optimistic in nature and focus on what they have. Conversely, those who view the glass as half empty are more pessimistic in nature and tend to focus on what they lack.

In my own life, I have found these principles to be most true. Each time I have had an idea that I got excited about and believed I could accomplish, circumstances presented themselves to allow me to turn my ideas into reality. When I unduly worried about something, it tended not to get better until I was able to focus on the solution rather than the problem. In all situations, my outlook largely determined what was happening around me.

I also find these principles true when I look at the many people that I have attracted into my life. The connections that you make with people are often based on having something in common. You are attracted to people on many different levels – mental, physical, emotional and spiritual – and one person may fill all or some of your wants and desires. I meet people so often in the most unlikely of places that have some connection with me that I have long since accepted that I am meant to meet them. I have attracted them into my life.

It is no coincidence that when couples meet, they are often doing things they enjoy at the same place at the same time. They were both attracted to the same situation. Each day you are placed in circumstances where you have something in common with those around you. Looking at what you gain from the experience will bring insight. Looking at what is lacking in the situation will make it far less pleasant an experience.

Why re-invent the wheel? Albert Schweitzer said: 'The greatest discovery of any generation, is that human beings can alter their lives by altering the attitudes of their minds.' By following his wisdom, you can adjust your attitudes to attract your desires into your life.

Attraction in action

What positive things have you attracted into your life? Think about an important experience when you got something that you really wanted. Try to think of an experience that was emotional in a happy and joyous way, such as getting your first

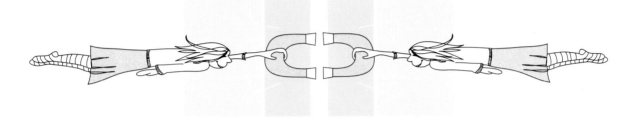

job or car. It could be something more personal such as the first relationship you were ever excited about. We often remember the first time we have done things in great detail. Think back on this experience, and try to recollect things as vividly as possible.

How old were you?
Where were you?
What were you wearing at the time?

How long had you wanted your desire to become a reality?

How often did you think about your desire?

Did you tell other people of your desire?

Did you imagine or see yourself in the situation as if it had already happened?

Did you think about it with great excitement?

When your desire finally became reality, did you then find more positive things seemed to occur soon after?

Set aside some personal time to think about each question. Sit in a comfortable space and take a few minutes to contemplate your answers.

Positive thoughts, emotions and expectations attract positive results. In this experience, your thoughts, emotions and actions were in harmony with your desires. The excitement stimulated your thoughts into imagining the possibility of having what you wanted. The end result was that you attracted the circumstances and situations to help you achieve your desires.

Look at the contrasts. Think about another situation when you thought you wanted something but did not get it; answer the same questions. Investigate how you were thinking at that moment and seek out those areas where you were focussed on the negative aspects of the situation.

Did you believe that you really deserved it, or were you sure that you really wanted it? According to the principles of how you attract things into your life, your thoughts or expectations were not aligned with your desire. Your old belief patterns may have prevented you from believing you deserved or could achieve what you wanted.

time to **assess**

Success in life is aided by believing in your own ability to accomplish goals, but is also influenced by having confidence in the way you tackle the task in hand. We can all benefit from a more positive outlook in some area. Looking at everything that is running smoothly, as well as things that are not working so well, can highlight contrasts in positive and negative approaches to situations.

By paying attention to what is occuring in the present, it is easier to let go of the old habits and ideas that formed your beliefs and attitudes in the past, and to develop new strategies of positive thinking to benefit your future. The Positive Behaviour Survey in this chapter reveals your current thoughts and feelings towards aspects of your day-to-day life. By finding out where you are at in this moment, you can see how your existing beliefs and attitudes affect your outlook. This survey analyses how your thought patterns impact on your approach to your daily habits, home life, career, relationships, and ability to lead the life you dream of.

Broken down into six sections, the Positive Behaviour Survey enables you to identify the areas that you most desire to change first. Each section of the survey relates to easy-to-use sections of the book that have simple exercises to inspire you along the way. Before beginning any project, it is always great to take a few minutes to think about what you would like to achieve in the process. If you are truly ready to see yourself as you are, use the information from the assessments as tools for growth. For once you shift your attitude about how you see the world, you will be able to see and experience all that you desire.

Your body image is the basis for your confidence in going out into the world and interacting with those around you. By reflecting on your attitudes about your appearance you can develop a better self-image. Likewise, it is easy to develop bad habits as part of your daily routine, which can become second nature. Taking a fresh look at how you approach daily chores can be invaluable.

When you are excited, you see the world through different eyes. Your vision is of hope and anticipation. As long as you are open to learning new things and having new experiences, you can gain enjoyment and satisfaction from whatever you do. All too often, however, in relationships and with work experiences, you shift your attention from that which you initially found exciting and made you happy, to those things in the situation that you do not like. This is particularly true of relationships. At the beginning, you see only the characteristics you want to see, but as you learn more about their personality, you begin to see things you do not agree with. When you focus your attention on areas of disagreement, you find more disagreement follows. By reflecting upon how you view others, you can learn to start consciously looking at the positives, and put fun back into your personal and professional life.

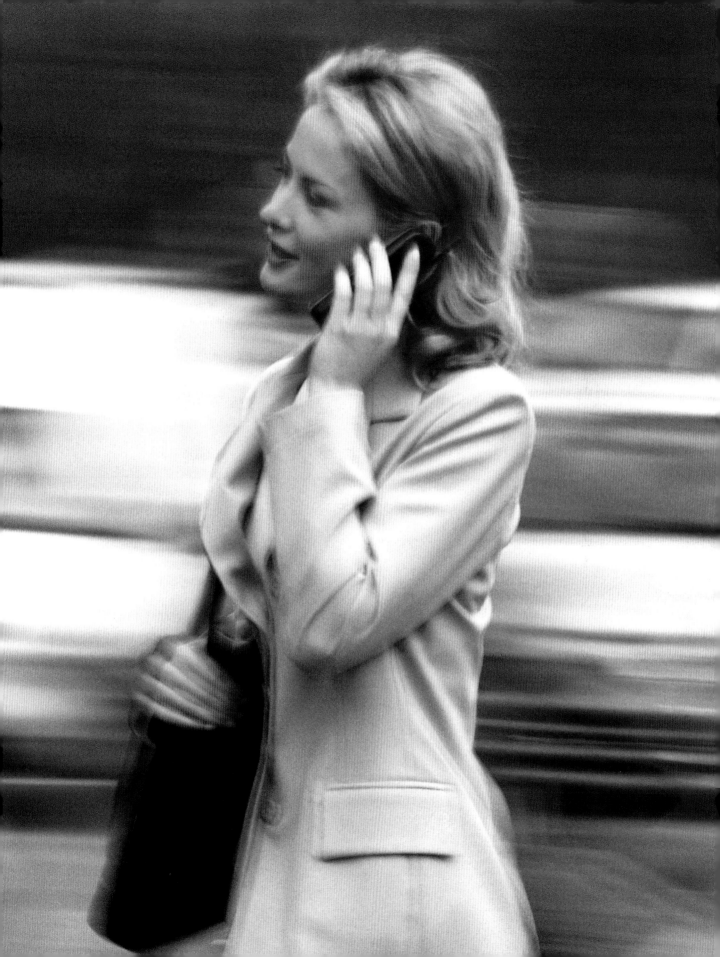

assess your **body consciousness**

From this day forward, be determined to see who you really are. Develop the habit of becoming conscious of what you are doing each moment to look after your magnificent machine. Looking after yourself shows appreciation for all that you are. Learn to reward yourself by doing something just for you.

1 When you think about your physical appearance, do you consider yourself:

a. your ideal shape
b. within reach of your ideal
c. out of shape
d. in dire need of help

2 When you walk past a mirror, do you:

a. stop and take a good look
b. glance and make adjustments
c. carry on without stopping
d. turn your head the other way

3 How happy are you with the amount of time you spend on your appearance:

a. very happy
b. quite happy
c. slightly unhappy
d. very unhappy

4 When you think about your appearance, does it make you feel:

a. proud
b. content
c. sometimes uncomfortable
d. always uncomfortable

5 How much time do you spend discussing your physical appearance with family and friends:

a. daily
b. weekly
c. every so often
d. never

6 To what extent does the media influence your ideas on physical appearance:

a. makes you want to be fitter
b. makes you want to pay more attention to your appearance
c. has no influence
d. makes you feel bad

7 Thinking about your physical body, list your best features. Start with those you desire to improve upon first:

Award yourself | 10 points for each A | 8 points for each B | 5 points for each C | 2 points for each D

60−50 points

You pay attention to your body and realise what is required to look as you desire. Your appearance is important to you and you always make a good impression on others. You appear confident, however, you may spend too much time worrying about your looks and be unduly influenced or competitive with those around you.

Make a list of the things about your appearance that do not satisfy you, starting with the one that displeases you most.

Keep yourself on track with the Maximise Your Appearance Positive Action Exercise on pages 42–3, but make sure your expectations are realistic.

49−32 points

You know that your appearance is not as you wish, but you have not really wanted to put in the effort required to change it up until now. You tend to start and stop fitness programmes and diets and sometimes feel guilty when you eat your food. You shy away from mirrors and tend not to want to see your weight.

Make a list of your vital statistics to take stock of who you really are.

height

weight

chest

waist

hips

Utilise the Sort Your Life 30-day Action Plan on pages 62–3 to stay conscious of how you are looking after your body.

31−12 points

You suffer from a poor self-image and hold your thoughts deep inside. You have a difficult time relaxing and often find yourself off in another world. You attempt to do something about your appearance but usually do not follow through. You have held these attitudes for a long time, but really want things to be different.

Make a list of your character traits to discover the you hidden deep inside. Start with all the positives first, such as generosity or humour.

Learn to use all your positive characteristics in every situation. The Positive Action Exercises on pages 42–5 will help to change improve your self image by taking action and rewarding results.

assess your **home comforts**

Coming to grips with maintaining a home can be daunting for even the best housekeeper. Learning to develop positive habits in organising your possessions can impact dramatically on how well you are able to utilise your space for enjoyment and relaxation, a vital necessity for peace of mind. By looking at the way you are currently using your home, you can gain more space and get more things done with less effort.

1 Is your home your favourite place to be?

a. always
b. frequently
c. sometimes
d. never

2 What percentage of your possessions do you find fit comfortably in their surroundings?

a. 100–75%
b. 74–50%
c. 49–25%
d. 24–0%

3 When did you last do something that inspired you in your own home?

a. within the last month
b. within the last six months
c. within the last year
d. cannot remember

4 Do you dream of a different type of living arrangement?

a. never
b. sometimes
c. frequently
d. always

5 Do you feel in control of your own space?

a. always
b. frequently
c. sometimes
d. never

6 Are the actions of other occupants in your household in harmony with yours?

a. always
b. frequently
c. sometimes
d. never

7 There are many elements to a room that make it feel comfortable. Think about your home and list those areas that you are happy with. Start with the things that you most enjoy.

Award yourself | 10 points for each A | 8 points for each B | 5 points for each C | 2 points for each D

60−50 points

You take pride in your home and appreciate spending time there. You are mostly organised and can easily find things when you need them. You are able to easily get around and use each room for its intended use. When you no longer require things, you find it easy to let go of them.

Make a list of any inspiring things that would make your home feel even better. If things become too routine we can stop appreciating them.

Concentrate on the areas of your home that will have the greatest impact on your day-to-day living. Chart your progress in tackling these problem areas on the Sort Your Life 30-day Action Plan on pages 62–3.

49−32 points

You have developed bad habits in your household activities, putting things off rather than immediately dealing with them. Often you cannot find things, causing you to be late. Sometimes you find it difficult to relax as many things need doing. There may be other people in the household who contribute to the problem.

Make a list of any irritating aspects of living in your home. You can set an action plan to implement change by acknowledging the problem areas.

Using the exercises in Take Charge of Your Space on pages 46–53, learn how to refresh and bring new energy into your home. Chart your success on the Sort Your Life 30-day Action Plan on pages 62–3.

31−12 points

Your home is not a place where you feel good about yourself. You do not know how to begin to sort it out as you have not been paying attention so things have built up around you. You cannot concentrate and are unable to relax. You do not use your home as a place to socialise. You spend a great deal of time worrying.

Make a list of the worst areas in your home. Start with the one element that makes you feel most uncomfortable.

Follow the step-by-step guide to Take Charge of Your Space on pages 46–53. Chart your progress in tackling these problem areas on the Sort Your Life 30-day Action Plan on pages 62–3.

assess your **positive power**

Gain an understanding of how your current ways of thinking impact on your life, learn to harness the power of positive thinking and boost your energy levels for dramatic results. When you are feeling positive, you attract more positive energy into your life. As a result, you are able to achieve more. By looking at how you have been thinking about situations in your own life, you can begin to shift your attitudes in a more positive direction. Just by shifting your attitude even slightly in the right direction, you will never go back to where you were.

1 In general, do you feel that things will work out for you?

a. always
b. frequently
c. sometimes
d. never

2 When you consider your day, in general, what percentage of your time is spent thinking about positive things?

a. 100–75%
b. 74–50%
c. 49–25%
d. 24–0%

3 When something good happens, how often do you tell someone else about it?

a. always
b. frequently
c. sometimes
d. never

4 Do you find more positive things happen as a result of sharing your good news with someone else?

a. always
b. frequently
c. sometimes
d. never

5 Have you ever noticed when you think about something, you start to hear more and more about it?

a. always
b. frequently
c. sometimes
d. never

6 Do you ever notice that when you feel good, you seem to be able to accomplish more?

a. always
b. frequently
c. sometimes
d. never

7 In the course of the day, we do many things. Think about your day and list those things that make you feel good. Start with the things that make you feel the best.

Award yourself | 10 points for each A | 8 points for each B | 5 points for each C | 2 points for each D

60−50 points

You are applying the principles of positive thinking most of the time and understand the benefits of doing so. You should harness this awareness and use this great energy-focussing ability you already possess to achieve success and happiness in all areas of your life.

Look at your list of daily activities that make you feel good. Now list all the other activities that you do during the day.

Apply your positivity to your own goals. Chart your personal growth and success with the Achieve Your Dreams 30-day Action Plan on pages 94–5.

49−32 points

You are randomly using your power of positive thinking during the course of your day to beneficial effect, but this is not consistent. In some instances, you may be holding on to old negative thought patterns in relation to achieving success in certain areas of your life.

Make a list of the daily activities that you feel good about but never seem to accomplish during the course of a normal day.

Using the Focus Your Attention Positive Action Exercise on pages 74–5, learn how to concentrate your energy on one goal at a time to achieve your objective.

31−12 points

You are aware that sometimes you get into a negative spiral and most things then seem to go from bad to worse. This awareness is the first step towards empowerment: now you can start to convert your negativity into a positive outlook on life.

Think about the one thing during the course of each day you want to change most. By changing this, you will dramatically improve the way you feel.

Using the Focus Your Attention Positive Action Exercise on pages 74–5, learn how to take small steps forward to achieve a positive end result. Slow and steady wins the race!

assess your **energy levels**

There are three integral ingredients that give us the vital life force energy that we require to stay alive. The food that we eat, the air that we breathe and the water that we drink are converted by our body into energy. Air and water are used by our cells to help them operate efficiently. The calories from the food we eat give us the physical stamina to be active. When all levels of our being are in harmony, our energy flows efficiently throughout our system. Noticing how your energy is during different times of the day, can help to see areas where your energy needs to be regulated.

1 Do you find that when you wake up in the morning, you are:

a. refreshed and ready to face the day
b. wanting a bit more sleep
c. needing some energy
d. unable to face the day

2 Do you have stamina throughout the day?

a. always
b. frequently
c. sometimes
d. never

3 Do you find that you can be influenced by other people's energy?

a. never
b. occasionally
c. sometimes
d. always

4 How often do you feel that your energy is scattered and not directed at a single purpose?

a. never
b. occasionally
c. sometimes
d. always

5 Do you feel like you look after your physical body?

a. always
b. frequently
c. sometimes
d. never

6 Do you pay attention to the foods you eat?

a. always
b. frequently
c. sometimes
d. never

7 Write down those things in the course of the day that seem to give you energy and make you feel good. Start with the ones you feel the best about.

Award yourself | 10 points for each A | 8 points for each B | 5 points for each C | 2 points for each D

60−50 points

You are looking after yourself and are aware that your lifestyle dictates how much stamina you have. Your body is receiving the nutrition it requires for all the activities you undertake. You have learned to regulate your energy and know how to relax.

List activities that give you energy
and make you feel good. Now list your favourite element to see the things that you can incorporate into other areas that need improvement.

Understanding the stimulation that gives you energy can help you to incorporate similar stimulation in other activities. Apply these positive motivators to activities in which you lack energy.

49−32 points

You do not always pay attention to your body. Physical signs of a lack of energy are headaches, muscle tension, dehydration and bad eating habits. Feeling tired and lacking energy can also result from not understanding how to regulate your energy, or failing to strike a balance between work and play.

Make a list of activities you enjoy
but suffer from an imbalance in your energy. Think about areas where you have too much energy to relax, or not enough to participate.

Using the Take a Walk on the Wild Side Positive Action Exercise on page 83, learn how to gain physical stamina and boost your energy.

31−12 points

You have experienced health problems, such as allergies or issues with food, making it difficult to gain energy. Your body is not providing the stamina to break the cycle. You feel overwhelmed at the amount of things vying for your attention, and it is difficult to get things done. You worry about your situation and cannot find a way forward.

Make a list of all the factors
you believe are causing your lack of energy and focus.

Take responsibility for each of these factors in order to gain control of your body. Practise the Regulate Your Energy Positive Action Exercise on pages 84–5 and become more aware of your body's signals.

assess your **relaxation levels**

We all need to achieve a balance between work and relaxation in order to have a continuous flow of energy throughout our bodies. When we are in a relaxed state, our body shows physical signs through lowered blood pressure and deeper breathing. Relaxation helps our bodies to revitalise our cells and conserves energy for when we need more physical stamina.

1 Are you able to relax during the time you set aside for yourself?

a. always
b. frequently
c. sometimes
d. never

2 Do you have too many thoughts that make it difficult to switch off?

a. always
b. frequently
c. sometimes
d. never

3 Do you plan relaxing periods into your schedule?

a. always
b. frequently
c. sometimes
d. never

4 Do you find that you have tense situations at home or at work?

a. never
b. sometimes
c. frequently
d. always

5 Do you find it difficult to let others take charge?

a. never
b. sometimes
c. frequently
d. always

6 Do you worry about the outcome of most situations?

a. never
b. sometimes
c. frequently
d. always

7 There are many different ways to kick back and relax. Think about the most relaxing people, places and activities in your life and list all three separately. Start with those that you feel most comfortable with.

People

Places

Activities

Award yourself | 10 points for each A | 8 points for each B | 5 points for each C | 2 points for each D

60−50 points

You have learnt some effective strategies to give your mind and body the relaxation it requires. There are situations in your life you find stressful and have fallen into the bad habit of expecting to find tension in them. By practising your relaxation skills before you enter into stressful situations, you will find all activities more relaxing.

Make a list of situations that cause you tension and note down exactly what it is that you dislike about them.

Using the techniques in the Calm Your Mind Positive Action Exercise on pages 122–3, learn how to let go of the need to control all situations. Notice how life becomes generally more relaxing.

49−32 points

You sometimes have difficulty relaxing and getting a good night's sleep. You have a tendency to spend a lot of time thinking and find it difficult to get your brain to switch off. You have a lot of nervous energy and find it difficult to concentrate on things over a long period of time.

Make a list of any worrying problems occupying your thoughts. For each problem, write down the first ten solutions that come to mind.

Learn to trust that your mind can deliver the solution to any problem if you think about it in the right way. Go back to the Solve Your Problems Positive Action Exercise on pages 90–1 to put your mind at rest.

31−12 points

You suffer from a lack of physical energy caused by your inability to switch off your thoughts. You are not very connected to what is going on around you and have a tendency to live inside your head. You are not very grounded. Your health, mental and emotional states may be affected by your difficulties in relaxing.

Make a list of any traumatic events that may have occurred. Think back to when you first started to suffer from stress to detect any possible causes.

In order to belong to the present, you must relinquish the past. Practise the Calm Your Mind Positive Action Exercise on pages 122–3 and release all your old worries and fears. Move confidently towards the future.

assess your **fun factor**

When was the last time you had a good giggle or took your shoes off and walked through the grass? Having fun in everything that you do is the ultimate goal of a happy and fulfilled life. Too often we get bogged down in our old habits and forget to put the childlike magic into each thing that we do.

1 Do you have a good sense of humour?

a. always
b. frequently
c. sometimes
d. never

2 Are you able to laugh at yourself?

a. always
b. frequently
c. sometimes
d. never

3 At what point of your day do you first start to laugh?

a. first thing
b. afternoon
c. evening
d. never

4 Do you ever do something because the mood strikes you?

a. always
b. frequently
c. sometimes
d. never

5 Do you have fun in your most important personal relationship?

a. always
b. frequently
c. sometimes
d. never

6 Are you stimulated by your chosen life path?

a. always
b. frequently
c. sometimes
d. never

7 Do you try new things? Make a list of the activities in which you have the most fun. Start with the best first. Then list any relationships that bring fun into your life. Start with the most enjoyable first.

Award yourself | 10 points for each A | 8 points for each B | 5 points for each C | 2 points for each D

60−50 points

You are easy going and do not take yourself too seriously. You tend to lose interest in your pursuits when things become too serious. You are the kind of person that people enjoy being around as you bring laughter with you, but may tend to sometimes be unreliable in your own pursuit of fun.

Make a list of situations and people that you need to take more seriously. Sometimes laughter can mask an inability to relate on a deeper level.

Go back to the Regulate Your Energy Positive Action Exercise on pages 84–5 to balance your fun side with your serious side, then tackle the Get the Buzz Positive Action Exercise on pages 114–15.

49−32 points

You know how to have a good time and are able to integrate fun activities into some parts of your life. You are sometimes willing to take a risk and are able to look at some situations from a fresh point of view. You may find certain activities more tedious than others and need to look towards your strengths in those situations.

Make a list of activities in your life that could do with a injecting a bit of spontaneity.

Take suggestions from the Get the Buzz Positive Action Exercise on pages 114–15 to add some new energy to an old situation.

31−12 points

You spend too much time looking at all the things you do not have in your life. You are very set in your ways and find it difficult to look at things from a different perspective. You are probably holding on to old traumas and need to have a dramatic shift of attitude. You are ready, willing and able to put some fun back in your life.

Consider the most important area of your life that needs a lighter touch. List five ways you could make the situation more fun.

Learn to create your own fun in life by practising all the Positive Action Exercises in the Have Fun chapter, which will help to bring joy to all your day-to-day situations.

time to assess **summary**

Each assessment in the Positive Behaviour Survey is intended to get you to look at your current habits and attitudes, which may affect how you feel towards your current lifestyle. You need to take time out to tune yourself back into the basics of paying attention to your thoughts and emotions.

Your emotions let you know how you feel on the inside. Sometimes they feel great, but sometimes they do not. By becoming aware, we learn that when we feel great, we are fulfilling our inner desires. When we feel bad about something, see how our thoughts are influencing the outcome of the situation.

If you look your responses to all of the surveys together, you may begin to see patterns that carry through from one area of your life to the next. When looked at as a whole, it may seem like an overwhelming amount of change is necessary to get where you want to be. In reality, change can be quite dramatic, or quite slow, depending on how willing you are simply to let go of old habits and ideas. Open up your heart to new ideas, and allow energy to flow efficiently throughout your body.

To achieve successfully the results you desire, you must believe that you can do it. Using all of the creative methods in the Achieve your Dreams chapter may help to stimulate new ways of approaching situations.

Each chapter includes methods that have been used successfully to change attitudes and behaviours that are no longer wanted. The more committed you are to wanting something better, the more aware you become of making the choices that make you feel better.

Starting with paying attention to your physical body, you can gain greater control of all of your senses to help you be in touch with your innermost dreams. Allowing yourself to experience fun and joy, because you are feeling that you are doing what is right for you in the moment, is to acknowledge that you hear your inner voice.

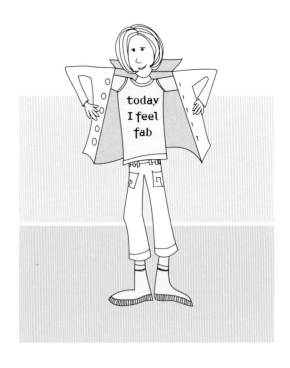

To use this book most effectively, I suggest that you prioritise your efforts, beginning with the area that is easiest to change. Rate all the following areas in order of ease and speed in achieving results, having looked at the outcome of your personal assessments. Start with the one that has the least emotional issues surrounding it, and that is more likely to be a problem through not paying attention to the issue.

- Physical health
- Physical appearance
- Living conditions
- Organising skills
- Positive attitude
- Looking at different ways of doing things
- Improving self confidence
- Relaxation
- Relationships
- Having fun

Release unwanted emotions

As you begin to see that you have the ability to change your behaviour by the way you think about situations, you gain confidence and know that you can change situations by looking at them in different ways. With this knowledge, you can begin to want to let go of old emotional issues that keep you in the past. Begin to tackle the situations on your list that may have developed over a longer period of time and be associated with past feelings. You can dispose of these feelings quite simply, when you decide you are ready to let them go. You do not have to spend any time dwelling on what the significance of it might have been in your life, you just simply have to say goodbye, forgive yourself and others for the past and let it go, because you are ready for something better.

Make the commitment

In everything you do, there must be an exchange of energy – some form of commitment that makes the work meaningful. Within Western cultures, an exchange of money makes a contract binding. Other cultures use a barter system, swapping goods or services for other goods or services. However, an exchange of energy can be anything that is done with the intention of completing the experience.

Keep a personal journal. Set aside thirty minutes each evening to write down the day's events and your thoughts and feelings. Let go of all that happened, without judging what occurred. The easiest way to do this is not to worry about how silly your writings sound or whether you use the best grammar or spelling. It can simply be thoughts, lists or literally whatever pops into your head and onto the page. Do not even bother to read it back. No one will ever see the contents of this journal and it is strictly a method of letting things go without emotion. For the first thirty days, do not go back and read any of the pages.

Make the conscious decision to feel better. There is no need to analyse the significance of releasing old habits or emotions, other than deciding how those things make you feel is no longer wanted in your life. Spending too much time thinking about what was, keeps you glued to the past. The more you are able to let go of things that happen daily, the easier it is to let go of the big things in some meaningful way. Once you are able to let go of that thought pattern, by writing it down, know that it is gone forever and release the old ways of thinking.

Enjoy the daily process. At the end of each thirty-minute session, take an extra five minutes to write down five things that you are grateful for having happened that day. It can be absolutely anything. After writing, close your book and go straight off to sleep.

sort your life

"The difference between what we do and what we are capable of
doing would suffice to solve most of the world's problems."
Muhatma Ghandi

We often need a kick up the backside to prompt us to change the things we
dislike about our lives. You may develop health issues that require a change in
lifestyle, indicating your old habits were detrimental to your well-being. You may
have emotional problems that lower your self-image and make it difficult to trust
your decision-making ability. Sometimes you just take on board too many things
and are unable to concentrate long enough on one project to take action. The end
result is that you become stuck in a rut and need some help to get back on track.

Before you can achieve your dreams for the future, you must sort out your
life in the present. Because you are a physical being, you cannot help but pay
attention to the physical reality of your life. If you have problems with your health,
the pain is difficult not to think about. If your living space is chaotic, the clutter
that you see daily is difficult not to think about. If you constantly run out of time
trying to get things done, the unfinished projects are difficult not to think about.

You spend much of your time focusing on what you do not want, such as
pain, chaos and confusion, so you get back more of the same. Taking action to
tackle areas you find problematic, will leave your mind free from all thoughts of
what you do not want. It is only by clearing the decks and getting on with your life,
that you can understand the limitless possibilities of all you can dream and achieve.

This chapter is aimed at tackling three areas that many of us struggle with
– how you feel about your body, how you live and work in the space you create,
and how you manage to organise your time and get things done. When you have
a clear mind, fit and healthy body and surroundings that are relaxing, there are
no obstacles to prevent you from thinking about and getting what you want.

It is best to start with the area that you believe is the easiest and quickest
to remedy. Something that you believe is achievable will get done. It also
indicates that there are fewer emotional issues associated with this area of your
life and the patterns will be easy to change. Issues with your living space can
often be tackled in a dedicated weekend and will instantly help you to see and
feel the difference. Remember that positive thoughts and emotions attract more
of the same, so after one success, the next area will seem within easier reach.

Take charge of your life. When you are in control, there are no excuses: you
are responsible for your every action. We often focus on the reasons why we cannot
do things to absolve ourselves of the responsibility. By dwelling on problems, you
cannot be thinking about solutions. It is only by focussing on solutions and taking
steps towards them, that positive outcomes can be achieved. An anonymous writer
once remarked that the road to elevated fortune is in elevated actions. I agree.

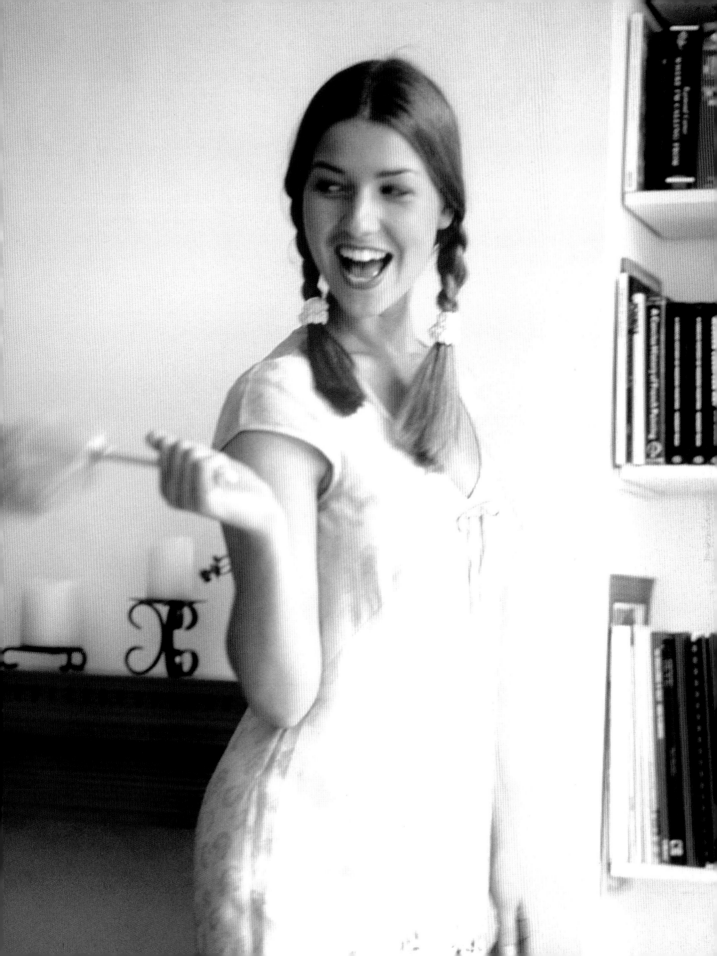

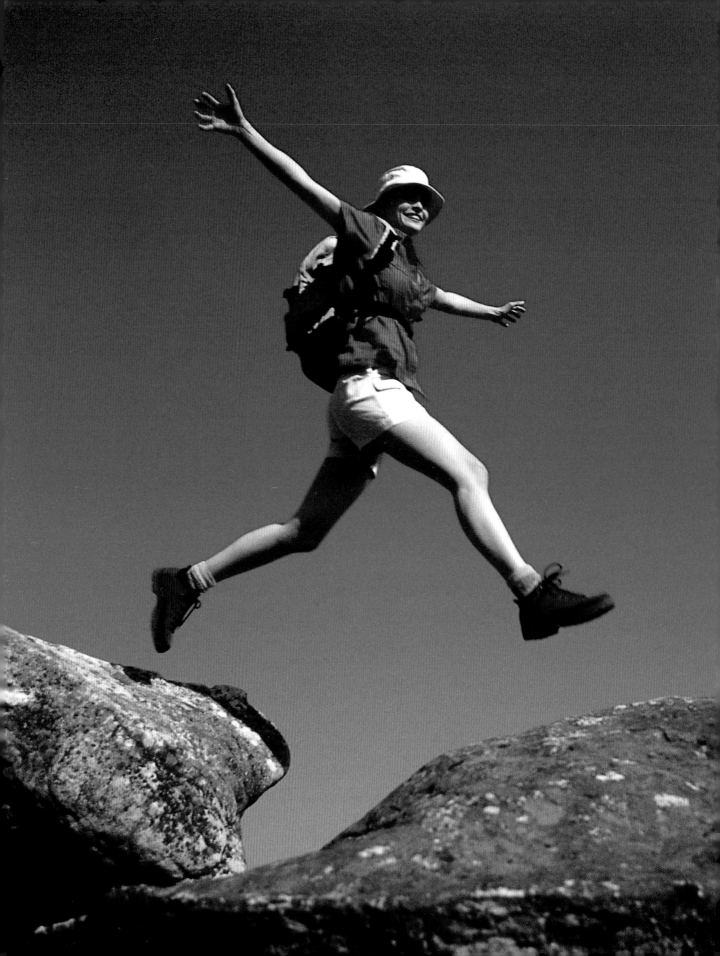

act now

The biggest obstacle to taking action is confusion, too many things competing for your attention at the same time. You often try to accomplish too many things at once and end up getting nothing done. Think about what you want to accomplish as you begin each part of your day. Without setting your intention, you do not signal your mind that you require all of your available mental energy to concentrate on accomplishing your desire.

Sheer determination, or simply focussing all of your attention on one thing, is a difficult force to beat. Look at any athlete that performs almost super-human feats and you will see how an individual's will can achieve more than most even dream. The power of their thoughts and emotions stimulate a physical response by producing adrenalin, which gives a sudden increase in physical strength. The body responds quickly to what is required.

Desire brings forth the determination to see clearly towards achieving your goals. No matter how many times you tell yourself that you need to take action over matters in your life, it is not until you truly want it for yourself, that you commit to action from your heart, where you know your personal truth. Once you open your heart to your intention, the process becomes a labour of love rather than a chore. When you feel joy, once again your body responds by producing endorphins that stimulate your brain and promotes a feeling of well-being.

When you begin your personal programme for change, you must set aside personal time, without distractions, to focus your energy and attention on getting what you want from the experience. There can be no excuses for interruptions, so carefully plan any additional help you may require to fulfil your commitments.

Throughout the work that you do, always think about your strong desire to succeed. Really, really want the end result and think about what it will be like when you have it. Be as creative as you can and use your imagination and all of your other senses to help you to get excited about the end result. Use whatever tools motivate you. Think about motivating people, locations, music and scents that inspire and uplift you to greater heights.

Each area has guided exercises to help you to release old habits, routines and thought patterns. You need to learn to forgive yourself and others for the disappointments that you have experienced. These feelings keep you tied to old events which you are doomed to repeat. Letting go of them feels as if a huge weight has been lifted from your heart and shoulders. Learning to be able to recognise your own accomplishments and not needing the praise of others to feel complete, is acknowledging your own power to get what you want.

The more you succeed, the greater belief you will have in your ability to utilise your thoughts for your highest good. The greater the faith that you develop that positive thoughts and emotions and belief will always end in positive results, the fewer times you will lapse back into disbelief. When you lapse into disbelief, you are no longer able to see the small signs of progress you have made.

gain control of your body

With a busy life, sometimes you to forget to look after yourself. Get reacquainted with your body to see where you are. Look at the daily actions you take, and how they affect your health. I believe you can change how you feel physically purely through the strength of your mind. You do not need fad diets, you just need to pay attention to your routines and habits and note any changes required to bring your body into a fit and harmonious state of being.

Step one

Become aware for the next 24/7. Tune into how you feel. For the next week, each evening before you go to bed, write down as much as you can remember about the following parts of your day:

How did you feel when you woke up?

Did you have enough energy for the day?

Did you feel anxious or tense at any time?

Did you feel relaxed, happy or laugh at any time?

Were you unable to concentrate at any time?

Did you eat at the same time each day?

Did you feel satisfied after eating your meals?

Did you take any physical exercise?

What time did you go to sleep?

Did you feel physically unwell at any time? If so, list the symptoms and time of day.

Did you have any personal treatments, such as a haircut or massage? If so, how often do you have them? If no, when did you last attend to your health or appearance?

Did you take any breaks during the day? If so, describe everything you did during your break times. If you were with others, what did you discuss?

Cause and effect

There is a cause and effect to every action you take. Reflect upon your answers and look at how the actions you took made you feel. Be aware of how your actions relate to your feelings. Take responsibility for the conscious choices you make.

Once you are able to see how your eating, drinking, sleeping and other daily habits impact on your health, you can change your attitudes and focus on feeling good. If you know that you require seven hours of sleep, three meals a day, and feel ill when you eat seafood, it would not be very sensible to eat seafood with regularity.

We all overindulge occasionally, but when it becomes a matter of course, as with all routines, we no longer see our habitual behaviour. You end up feeling bad more often than not, and it is not until the moment when you want to feel better that things change. In addiction programmes, this is described as hitting rock bottom. But why wait to feel that bad when you can choose to feel better?

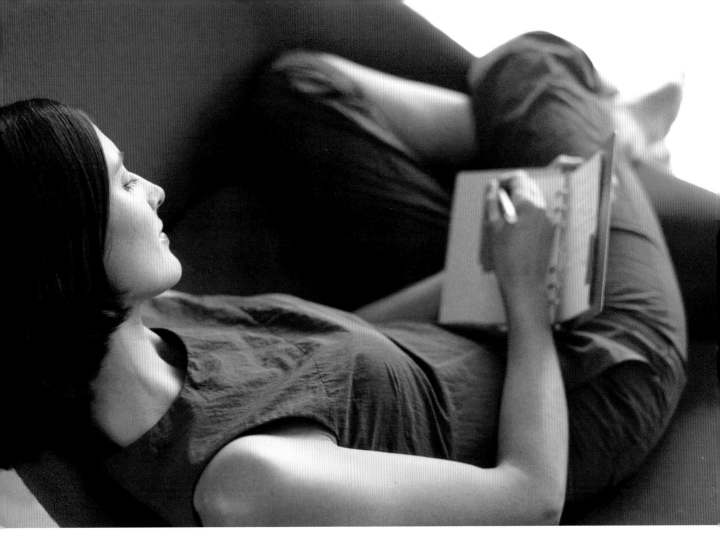

Step two

Changing your actions makes you aware of when you need to nourish your body and soul; changing your thoughts and attitudes gets you quicker results. Your thoughts towards your daily activities also effect how your body responds.

Write down what you were thinking about when you engaged in the following activities. Note all that immediately comes to mind:

| What did you think about first thing in the day?

| What did you think about whilst at work?

| What did you think about in the evenings?

| What were your thoughts upon going to bed?

| Did you dream? Write down any you remember.

Cause and effect

You have looked at how your actions affect your physical health and well-being. Take another look at the list in Step One to see if you can detect any ways in which your thoughts affect your health.

I have found that people who have difficulty with food intolerances or weight problems, think about food in a negative way. If you believe that the food you eat will cause an intolerant response, or will make you gain weight, the odds are quite high that it will. If, however, you simply think that the food you eat will nourish each and every cell of your body and give you the stamina that you require before you eat each meal, by changing from a negative thought to a positive thought, you will attract nourishment and stamina and will be able to change your physical condition.

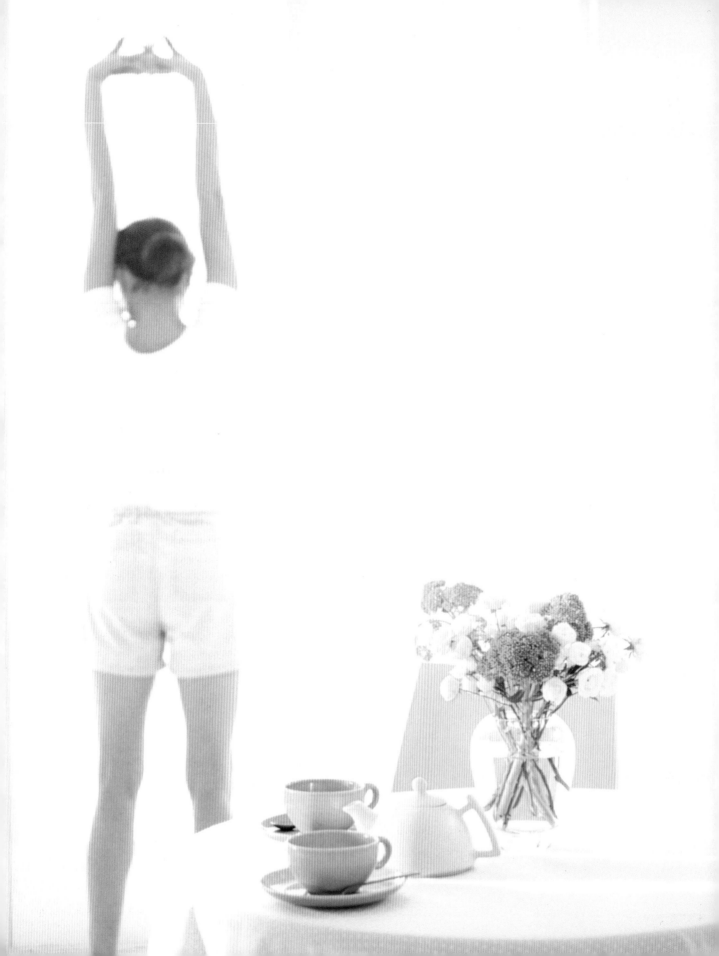

feel better every day

If your physical condition is getting in the way of achieving your dreams, it is important to stick to a programme of consciously choosing to feel better each day. Understanding that your thoughts are powerful attractors, by changing what you think about when you experience physical discomfort, you can pave the way towards feeling better.

Learn to heal

In my Reiki practice as a teacher, I have realised that everyone has the capacity to be a healer. Reiki is an ancient healing method that requires prolonged study with a Reiki Master. There are, however, simple healing techniques that you can use daily, or whenever needed, to consciously change how you feel physically. One of the most important parts of this healing tradition, is in the Reiki Principles:

- Just for today, do not worry
- Just for today, do not hold on to anger
- Just for today, honour your parents, teachers and elders
- Just for today, earn your living honestly
- Just for today, show gratitude to all living beings

We all can summon the strength and determination for one day to accomplish anything we reasonably believe we can achieve. Taking one day at a time keeps you focussed in the present moment, enabling you to see the fruits of your actions take hold.

Tune into your body

Before you can heal, you must tune into the signs your body gives you on a daily basis. Your inner guidance makes it really easy to know when you are on the right path to achieving your innermost desires. Whenever you are on track, you are rewarded by feeling good – the right amount of energy, fine physical appearance and body condition. The more appreciative and joyous you are of the process, the better you feel.

Whenever you are feeling bad, your guidance is telling you, in that moment, you are not moving forward. Your thoughts and emotions are holding you back. In noticing the physical symptoms of disease, you can use this indicator to change how you may be thinking at the time you are experiencing discomfort. In most circumstances, it is the worry or attention that you pay to the feeling that perpetuates it. Simply by doing something that feels better, you are consciously taking an action to advance and improve the situation.

Each time you change the way you react to a situation, you change your response forever. If, for example, each time you attend a meeting you experience an upset stomach, by changing that reaction just once, your expectations have been altered. In every situation you enter, you have a choice. By consciously choosing the option to feel better, you begin to understand that you have the power to focus your attention on the things that you want – a healthier, happier life – rather than living an experience that makes you feel bad.

maximise your appearance

>> positive action exercise

Much of how you feel about your physical appearance is determined through childhood, when looking 'average' feels safe. But for all those 'average' people in the middle, there are necessarily those on either end of the spectrum. Height, bone structure, ethnic features, wearing glasses, being right or left handed, or having ginger hair can make you stand out from the crowd.

Many pressures can lead you to seek the safer option of blending into the middle and can often be the result of the relationship with your parents and siblings. Where you fall in the pecking order of your family structure often determines whether you become an individualist or part of the pack.

By blending in rather than celebrating your uniqueness, you either over- or undercompensate to reach the middle. When you lower your expectations to fit into the mainstream, you often hold a deep resentment for not achieving all that you believed you could achieve. When you overcompensate and act out to be heard, you may achieve what you want, but it will be a painful process.

Trying too hard to be something that you are not will never make you feel good physically and can often feel like a pushing/pulling sensation within. As you develop your awareness of what your body is telling you, remind yourself to always be who you are inside.

Those who regard their uniqueness as an attribute, or think positively about their differences, are appreciating their special gift. They often lead by example and lift others to greater heights.

Make a list of those people who stand out most in your mind, and once you have done that, think about the things that make them most memorable.

_____   _____
_____   _____
_____   _____

When you look back over your list, you may find that it is the inner qualities of people that matter most.

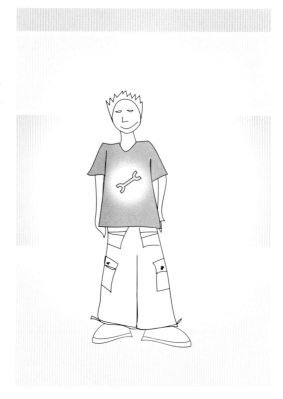

Inner glow toolkit

Your appearance is the outward reflection of how you view yourself in the moment. There are three things that make up someone's appearance: the physical traits that you cannot change; what you choose to look like through clothing and other personal expressions, such as hair and makeup, which you can alter by situation; and the way you look after your body, reflected in your weight, complexion and posture, which can be altered by your thoughts and actions. But have you ever noticed how certain people seem to have another quality, an inner glow that emanates light from within the body? People in love often have it as do many pregnant women or those who seem to have an innate love of life.

Whenever we open our hearts, we allow this inner glow to be seen by others. All emotions that stimulate the heart can help to change our appearance. Look at any proud couple who beam at the achievements of their children. Their love is reflected in their eyes – the windows of the soul. You do not notice what they are wearing, but what is striking is the outward reflection of their love for their offspring. You can easily see the impact of your inner glow by trying a quick experiment. Stand in front of a mirror and see what looks better – you with a smile on your face or you with a frown. Being positive affects your appearance in a more meaningful way than what you wear and attracts those people with the same depth of feeling into your life.

Your inner glow shines brightest when you speak, act and feel from your heart. In everything you do, you can change your appearance by choosing to start each segment of your day with a joyous attitude and an open heart. Try it and see how it works for you.

Just like applying a fake tan, you can get an instant inner glow by bringing your body into a state of joy. Assemble your own mental toolkit that you can use to bring out your inner glow in minutes.

Here are some suggestions that may work for you.

- Think about someone you love very much

- Think about someone who inspires you

- Think about making a gift to someone because you care about them. Take time to choose mentally the perfect gift, and imagine what it would be like to give it to them

- Imagine a location that you find peaceful and go there in your mind

- Sing your favourite uplifting song in your mind

- Tell yourself your favourite joke

- Flirt with a baby in your mind

- Think of stroking your pet

List any additional people, places or things that you love to add to your own personal toolkit that will bring out your inner glow.

Before you begin getting dressed for the day, take a few minutes to run through your mental toolkit to bring out your inner glow.

dress for success

How you dress tells the world a lot about the way you view yourself. In each role that you take on during the course of your day, you must judge what is appropriate. Attending a high-powered corporate meeting in jeans may be acceptable in some companies but not others. Turning up in fancy dress at a black-tie affair may be just plain embarrassing. Either way you need to understand the rules of the game to make appropriate choices.

Taking the time to think about the impact your clothing may have in each situation shows that you are actively thinking about how you express yourself. It means you are paying attention to what is going on around you. It also means that you will learn by your actions.

There are extremes in every situation: some of us spend too much time worrying, whereas others spend no time at all, appearing as if they do not care. The more confident you feel, the greater an awareness you will have about what is appropriate.

Look at the situations in your life that you wish to improve upon and see what signals you are giving off to those around you. Your clothing displays your feelings towards what you are engaged in. If your love life has lost its spark, you may find that you no longer make the effort to look good for your partner. If you are not taken seriously in some situations, perhaps your outward appearance might benefit from a re-think.

Consider the statement your clothing makes about you in the following areas of your life. Write down how much time you spend preparing and dressing for the following occasions and what you are most likely to wear.

- In the office or out at a meeting
- Working from home
- At home alone or with your family
- Out for a romantic dinner with your partner
- Out for a night with friends
- Visiting family or friends

It is easy to continually resort to a uniform – a generic look that says 'this is who I am'. If this suits your lifestyle and works for you, continue. Sometimes, however, you can get into the habit of not bothering. This can and does effect how you interact socially with others. A shift in attitude can dramatically alter the situation.

Now look at your clothing and assess how your wardrobe makes you feel. List how much of your clothing fits into the following categories:

- comfortable and relaxed
- capable and professional
- young and fun
- more mature
- serious and sombre
- sexy

Is the proportion of clothing in each category representative of your current lifestyle? As you experience new things, your requirements change. Most of us are guilty of hanging on to things way past the time that they are appropriate to our current situation. Your body shape changes, you grow older and you must keep up with the times. Letting go of the old image of yourself will feel a lot better: you will see yourself for who you are now.

Feel good toolkit

We all have special items of clothing, jewellery or a scent that makes us feel like a million dollars. Do you feel pretty in pink? Do you feel passionate in red? Do you feel innocent in curls or sophisticated with an updo? Does the smell of gardenias bring you to a higher place?

Colour and fragrance can enhance your mood and even change how you feel physically. More and more institutions such as offices, hospitals and shopping complexes are paying great attention to regulating our moods through colour and scent.

Put together a feel good toolkit that you can use to boost your self esteem and help you to get what you want out of each situation. We all react to colours differently: shades that are relaxing to some may cause agitation in others. Look at the colours you are attracted to and see how you can use them daily to enhance how you look and feel. The colours listed below are said to have the following properties:

Red is associated with strength and vitality, but is also seen as passionate and angry. It is a colour that helps us to take action and feel grounded, but those with high blood pressure or prone to anger should stay away from this colour.

Orange is associated with creative energy. It can help those lacking energy or feeling depressed.

Yellow is associated with the sun. A stimulating and positive colour. If you do not get enough daylight, wearing yellow is the next best thing.

Green is associated with nature and relaxation, as well as jealousy and envy. Located at the centre of the spectrum, it represents balance, although wearers of green may be suffering from some emotional imbalance.

Blue is associated with peace and tranquillity. Used in places requiring a calm atmosphere. Some shades of blue can aggravate depression.

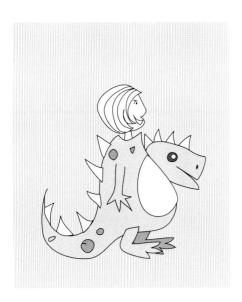

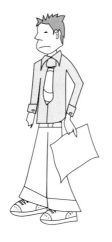

Indigo is associated with the night sky. It combines the properties of both blue and violet, and can help to clear your mind. If you are drawn to this colour, it may indicate that you need to relax.

Violet is associated with spirituality and inspiration. A colour that helps balance how you feel about yourself and encourages you to be accepting of your inner qualities. Wear violet when you need some self confidence.

take charge of your space

How you live in your home is a reflection of how well you are doing in your life. It is not just the material things you acquire that indicate your contentment with the path you have chosen, it is also the quality of your space and how you utilise it.

Many people's homes are filled with material possessions purchased as a result of what they desired at a particular point in time. They represent an achievement at a specific moment. As you experience more things in life, you continue to want new things, so your possessions build up without you seeing it happen. As a result, your material things outgrow your space. There are a number of tell-tale signs. Look at some of the common indicators and see how many you can relate to:

| You spend quite a bit of time looking for lost items. This situation causes you some stress

| When you walk into your house you experience a loss of energy. You feel drained

| You find it hard to focus on getting things done around your house. There seems to be so much to do, you do not know where to start

| Certain rooms are uncomfortable to be in, perhaps due to excessive paperwork that needs to be done or excess junk that is stored here

| In some areas of your home, you have difficulty with relationships. This leads to tension

| You do not enjoy socialising in your own space

All of these feelings are signals that something is unbalanced in your home and you need to become more aware of what is going on around you. In some cases, your material possessions may be holding you back. When you are confronted by areas of your home that seem out of control, you can have a very physical and emotional reaction, such as a loss of energy, lack of attention and stress.

The solution can be as simple as focusing your energy and paying attention to your surroundings. If you find that you lose your keys each day, you must become aware of the physical state of the area around where you lose them. Does your handbag need to be tidied? Does you need to clear your desk or dressing table? Become aware of the pattern.

If you are physically prevented from getting the things that you want in your home, then it is high time for a good sort out. If you often have to climb over one object to reach something else, the odds are that you will eventually trip over the obstacle, causing you to pay attention to the situation. You must then learn to let go of things that no longer serve a function.

Explore ways of letting go of all unwanted possessions and utilising your space to its full potential. Learning to discriminate is a simple process of seeking out the things that make you happy right now. If you appreciate and use an item, then it is an important part of your surroundings. If not, it is time to say goodbye.

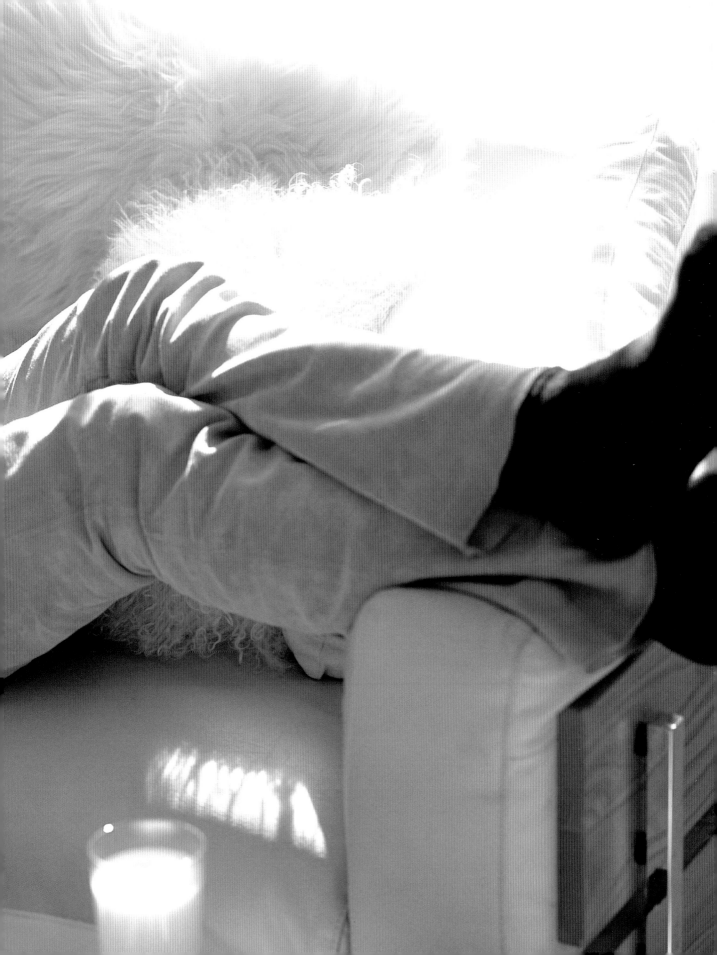

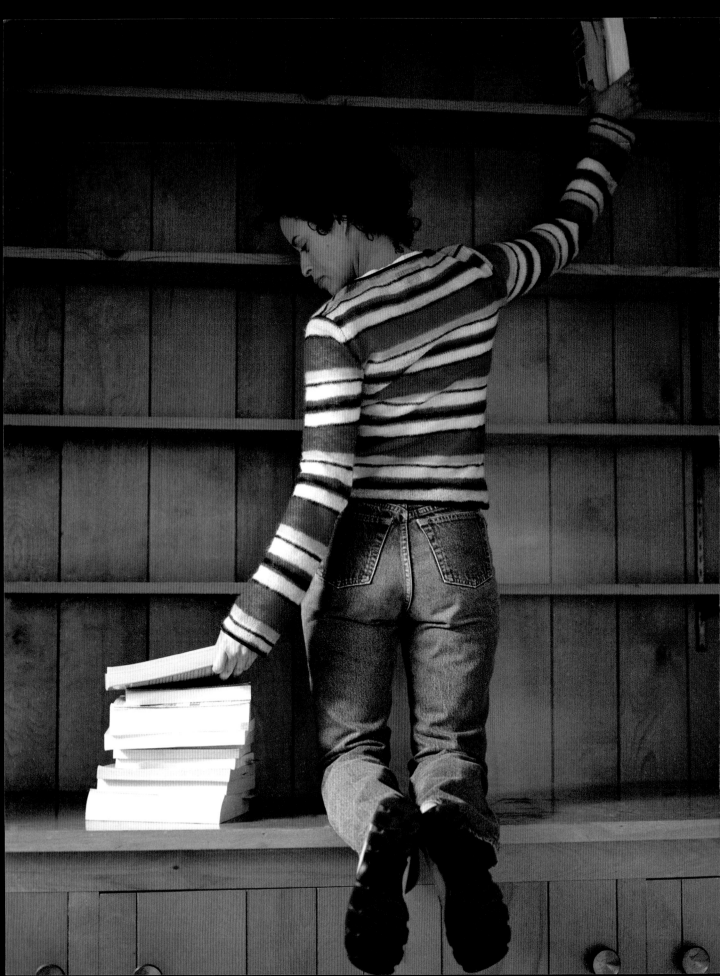

learn to discriminate

Through my experiences helping people to achieve a more harmonious home, I have found that, when space becomes a premium, it is easy to jettison 25 percent of what you own, that is items you have not looked at or used in a long time. Given the choice of ditching a few items that are surplus to requirements and enjoying more space or holding on to everything whether it is used or not and feeling cramped, most choose to have more space.

Most people hunger for more space. As you continue to buy things that you use and enjoy in the present, you are confronted with the many things you have purchased in the past. If the things you previously bought have hardly ever been used, you feel guilty at your extravagance, so you hold on to them with the determination to use them in the future. Why not be honest and confront the present? Live life to its fullest advantage.

Learning to discriminate is considering the options and making the choice that feels best in the situation. Try this simple exercise to see how quickly you can reduce the clutter in a problematic area of your home, without getting rid of anything but the junk. Allow yourself 15 minutes to get the job done:

Get rid of all junk paper. Recycle any newspapers, magazines and junk mail

Get rid of all empty containers. Recycle any aluminium cans, plastic bottles and cardboard

Put everything back in its place. Key items are clothing, CDs, other media and paperwork

This will make your space feel better immediately as less things are fighting for your attention when the junk is removed from the equation.

Now that you are able to look at your space with less clutter, you can start to use the discrimination process to decide what stays and what goes. To lighten the load by 25 percent, it is easiest to let go of those things that really no longer have a part to play in your current lifestyle. Pick the relevant categories for the room you are working to de-clutter and intend to let go of objects that you no longer use.

Furniture

Appliances

Clothes

CDs, tapes, records, videos and books

Souvenirs, photographs and sentimental objects

Hobbies, leisure and crafts

After letting go of things and freeing up space, spend some time thinking about how you feel in the room now. Do you have more energy or focus? Are you feeling more relaxed? This uplifting feeling of having shed some of the surplus weight will make it easier to continue with the process of paying attention to how things feel.

Now imagine how you would like your space to look and feel, and work towards your dream.

break down the barriers

Too many times in life you become stuck with the reality of a situation. You look at your house, with all of its walls intact, and feel hemmed in; all you can see is what is in front of you. Great architects and designers are visionaries, as they are able to see a space in all of its glorious potential. They do not see walls as barriers. As experience has proven, barriers can be broken down.

Consider any area of your home that presents a barrier. Look at furniture arrangements that may be barriers to communication, any items that are barriers to light, clutter that forms a barrier to access, or objects in your personal space that are a barrier to intimacy. Anything that gets in the way of allowing you to use your space for its intended use needs to be addressed.

Your home, whether rented or purchased, is most often the biggest investment that you will make in your life. As house prices escalate, it is more important than ever to make sure that your investment is being maximised. You work in order to enjoy life's comforts, recharge your physical body and reach your full potential.

Make a list of the areas of your home where there is most emotional conflict, starting with the worst room. Look at the physical configuration of the room now and then try to think back to when you first moved into the space. How did it feel when the room was a blank canvas? Back then you probably dreamed of how the space could be, of its potential. What got in the way? Write down all of things in the room that no longer fit your original dream. If you live in a household with others, get everyone in the house to share their points of view.

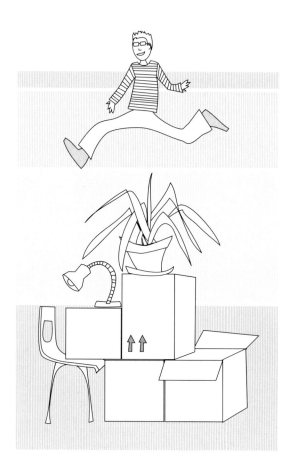

In all relationships, whether between members of your family, in your social or work environments, holding on to feelings means they are never expressed and resolved. This prevents you from living in the present moment. You are constantly confronted with past issues that block the way for effectively achieving all that you want in the present. By removing the physical barriers, you are often able to release the communication blockages as well.

Your mind is your most powerful tool for getting what you want. According to the universal truth of 'like attracts like', you attract whatever you are thinking. Do not waste this precious resource thinking about what you do not want, or you will get more of the same. Change the emphasis of your thinking to what you would like to happen, and set the wheels in motion to get the job done.

Think back to the moment you saw your home for the first time. Which elements attracted you to move there? Have you made the most of each of those elements? Do the rooms seem as large as they first did, or have you filled them so full of stuff that they no longer feel spacious?

When you first move into your home, you set up the rooms as you think they will be used. Surprisingly, most people only make a few changes after that. Maybe every five to ten years you will give a room a coat of paint to freshen things up, but you become comfortable with the familiarity, knowing where things ought to be, and rarely move on from there.

All too often, you stop seeing what is going on around you as it becomes too familiar; this commonly happens when things become routine. A room that once served as a guest bedroom can become a repository for unwanted junk. Family members may leave the home to start their own life, yet their room remains frozen in the past. Sometimes a communal living space, like the kitchen, turn into a dumping ground for things that are never put away. Frequently, you find that your lifestyle has changed and rooms that were once used often, like the formal dining room, are now only occupied on a very few occasions.

Make a list of all of the rooms in your home, including conservatories, lofts, cellars and any outbuildings. Against each room, write down how often the room is used:

Once you have completed your list, write down which activities you conduct in each room. If the room is used for storage or houses clutter, write down what is currently stored in that room.

Now make a list of all the things that you do on the run, using whatever space is available. This might include pastimes, such as painting and crafts, office work and even finding a personal space to relax and read a book.

Think about where you would like to be in your home. Replace under-used rooms with spaces that can dramatically impact on how you are able to accomplish your work or achieve your dreams. Look at ways of updating your independent children's rooms and make them inviting for guests to stay. Create a library on a large landing that may have just been accumulating junk. Open up your space for new experiences. Find a place to appreciate your passions.

Use your imagination to envisage your idea of a perfect living space. In this space, there is room for everything that you love having around and all those things that you use to make your life run smoothly.

review your space

>> positive action exercise

When your attention wains from what is going on in your own home, things can begin to build up without you even noticing. Often the situation needs to reach crisis point before you realise that you must take action. It can be something as annoying as never being able to find your keys, or a more serious problem like tripping over items that are never tidied away and put back in an appropriate place.

The purpose of this Positive Action Exercise is to look objectively at each room in your house from a different perspective. Set aside an hour of uninterrupted time when you can work through this exercise, then find a comfortable place for you to sit and write.

Sit with your feet on the ground and your spine pressed against the back of a chair. Close your eyes and take a deep breath in, breathing from your diaphragm but keeping your shoulders from moving. Exhale to the count of seven. Do this two more times.

Imagine that you are going off on holiday to your favourite destination where you have rented a holiday retreat. When you arrive, you are surprised to find that your vacation house is absolutely identical to your home in every detail – from the layout of the furniture to the untidied clothes, unwashed dishes and incomplete paperwork.

You have been asked by the management company of the holiday retreat to write a report on the condition of the house, and how it lived up to being a retreat. It is often easier to look at things when we are able to disconnect from the experience. Rather than looking at all the excuses of why your house may not be ideal, just looking at what it is and writing down what you see, can inspire you to think of ways of making it better. Answer the following questions:

| What was your initial impression of the house?

| Was it well looked after?

| Was it easy to get around?

| Did it feel spacious, light and cheerful?

| What were the most comfortable rooms?

| Why were they comfortable?

| Did you find things easily?

| Did you have everything you required?

| Did you find places to relax?

| Would you come back?

| How much would you pay to rent it for a week?

| Add any suggestions to improve your stay

Become the manager of your space and take action on the ways to improve your stay! Your home can be your retreat each day, by choosing to have things that you want and bring you pleasure, arranged in a way that makes you comfortable.

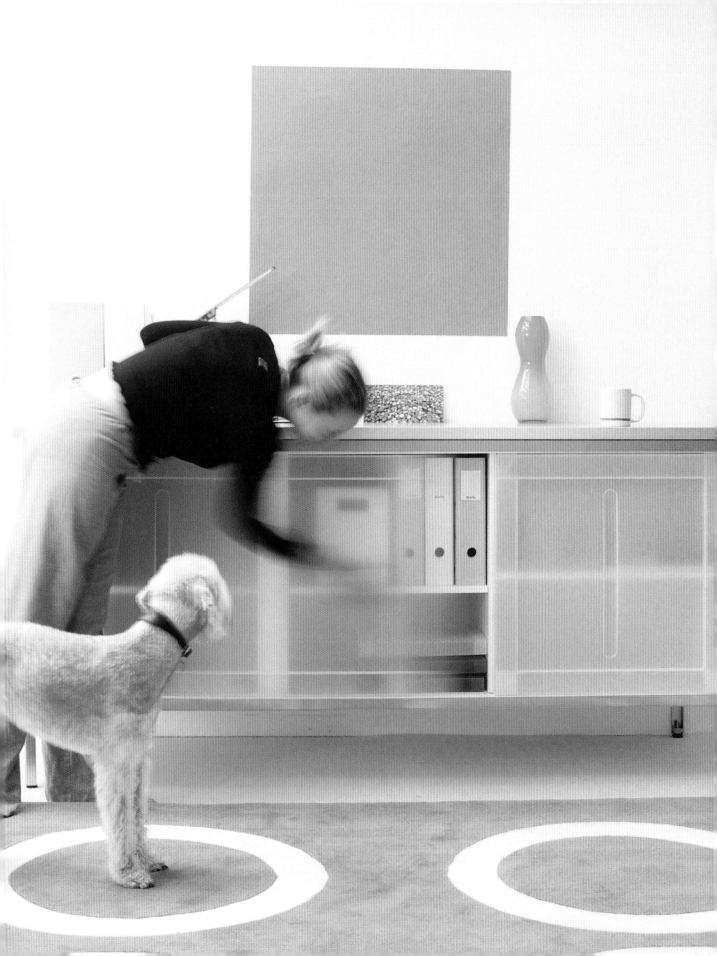

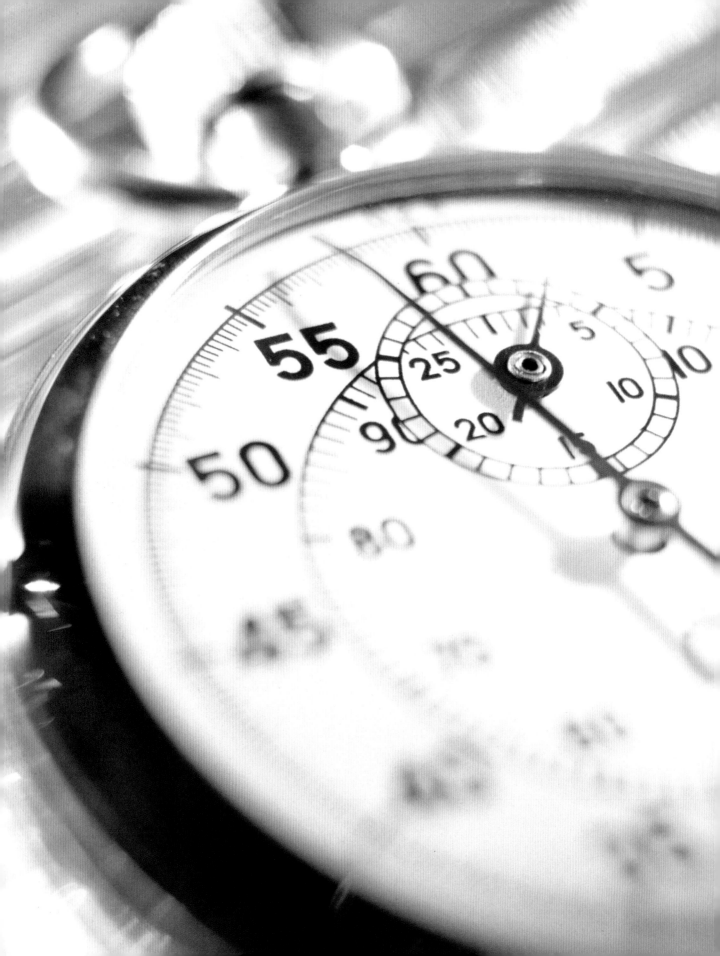

rule your time

Getting to grips with organising a busy life can make all the difference to how much you are able to accomplish on a daily basis. How you feel about yourself – your self esteem – is built, in part, on how you view your own achievements relative to your goals.

When you do all that you set out to do each day, you feel satisfied and good about yourself, as you are able to make things happen. By focussing your attention on what you want, you are inspired towards reaching your goal. Thinking about what you want, gets results. Getting enthusiastic about it, gets it more quickly.

We all feel frustrated if we are unable to get things done when they are needed, which has a knock-on effect as things build up around us. Usually, the cause of being unable to complete a task is distraction – thinking of too many things at the same time and being unable to focus – which results in not giving your undivided attention to what you want in the moment. All too often you put the blame on others as an excuse for being distracted from the task at hand. The reality is that nothing can distract you from what you really want.

Each time you think about something, you summons more information relative to that thought. The more thoughts you have about things that are irrelevant to what you are trying to achieve, the more information you get, which can lead to confusion and the inability to take action. The worse you feel about a situation, the more

difficult it becomes. We can all find examples of things that we do not enjoy doing that really become a chore and seem to take a long time to complete.

There will always be some things that you enjoy doing more than others, either through a sense of personal satisfaction or gained from the praise of others. You are more likely to be passionate about things that you hold dear to your heart, therefore you achieve these things more easily. However, you still have to do those things that you have come to dislike. By simply looking at how you approach the things that seem to take more time than you would like, you can consciously change your thoughts and attitudes to get things done more joyfully and efficiently.

All of your behaviour is learned over time and through experience. We all get into habits that simply become the routine way that we do things. You simply stop thinking so much about what you want to do and lose interest. It is like being on autopilot. Not only is it boring, as you are not truly connected to what is going on, but you can easily be swept away by events and circumstances and find it difficult to get things done.

The only way to rule time is to think in advance of each experience and what you want to get out of it. Bear this in mind throughout and then, once it is all over, clock the results. As you begin to expect to get things done, you will manage to get them done.

take away the pressure

Each day you are faced with the many responsibilities that are required to maintain your existence. As well as looking after yourself, you may also have the responsibility of bringing up a family. Juggling work-related responsibilities with your home and social obligations can make it difficult to get things done and leaves little time for your physical body to gain the relaxation it requires for balance.

How you think about the things you want to get done in a day, can dramatically impact on how long it takes you to get them done. Your desires, or wants, propel you forward towards achieving your goals. When you feel the need for something, however, you have shifted the emphasis from what you *want* to what you *lack*. There is a tremendous difference in how this makes you feel. Wanting is exciting. Needing is a pressure. What feels better, excitement or pressure?

By analysing how you feel about the things you do during the course of a normal day, you will gain an understanding of how your attitude affects the time it takes to get each thing done. Consider each activity listed here. Think about whether you feel that you need to do it or actively want to do it. Judge how you feel about each activity on the basis of how you most often feel about it.

Next, look at the items in your 'to do' list and think about how much time you spend trying to complete each task. Think about how you feel whilst you are doing this activity. Write down any activities that you tend to avoid doing as well as things that you never seem to accomplish.

Activity	Need	Want
Cooking a meal	☐	☐
Eating a meal	☐	☐
Doing housework	☐	☐
Working in the garden	☐	☐
Shopping for food and household items	☐	☐
Shopping for clothes	☐	☐
Attending to household finances	☐	☐
Conducting business by telephone	☐	☐
Socialising with friends	☐	☐
Talking with friends on the telephone	☐	☐
Working in your current job	☐	☐
Attending business meetings	☐	☐
Staying on top of office paperwork	☐	☐
Participating in sports or going to the gym	☐	☐
Going for a hair or beauty treatment	☐	☐

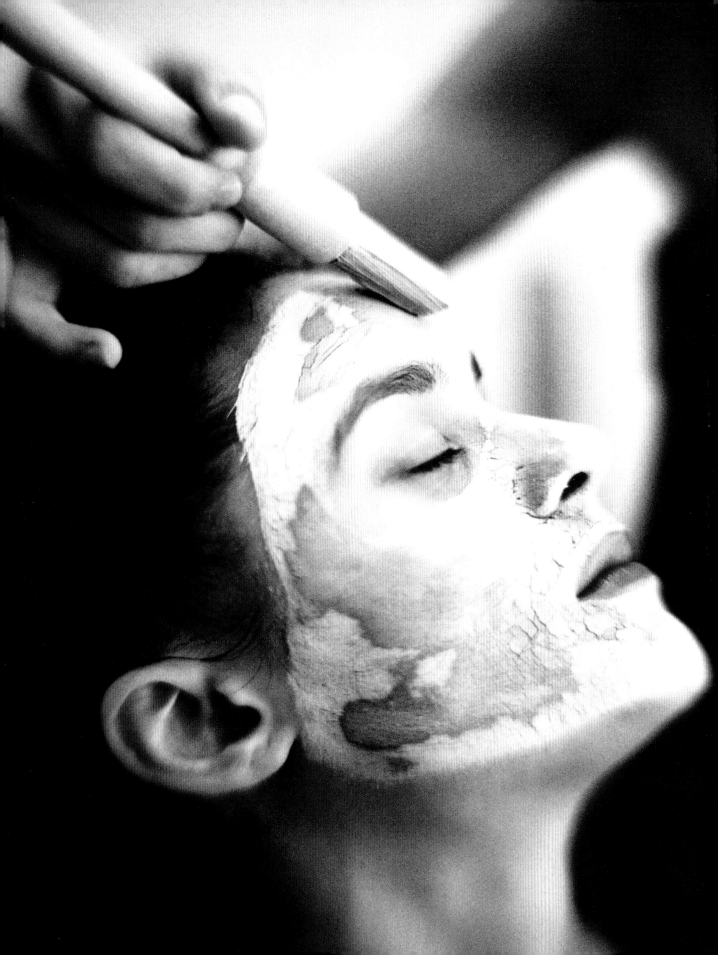

make time fly by having fun

>> positive action exercise

When you look at the things you do that take the least amount of time and effort, you will always find them to be the things that you actively enjoy and want to do. Your desire for the end result makes the effort worthwhile.

Think back to desperately wanting an ice cream on a really hot summer's day and going out to get it. Your excitement at the anticipation of that cool, sweet treat probably made the outing more of an adventure. Now compare that feeling with how you approach your weekly trip to the supermarket.

Look at anything that you feel a *need* to do, rather than a *desire*, and see if it feels more like a chore. The way you enter into each daily activity will determine the amount of time that the task will take. Before you start each project, you must take a few minutes to think about what you want to achieve in the time allowed. Making a list is always helpful in focussing your mind on the desired result. If, for example, you want to write a report, you may think about the following:

I want to write a report about four pages long

I want the report to be clear, concise and to the point

It feels good when the words flow and writing the report is effortless

I am excited at this opportunity to share my point of view

I like it when my ideas are understood

Focussing on the task in hand and more importantly, deciding what it is that you want to gain from the experience – whether in material or emotional terms – will help to speed things along.

This approach also works for more routine tasks around the house, such as doing the laundry. By appreciating the benefits of accomplishing this otherwise mundane task, you will experience how much better it feels when you think about a positive result.

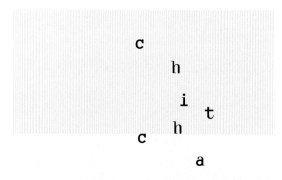

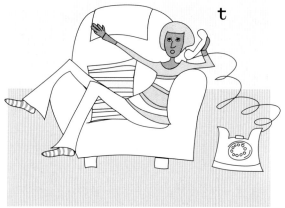

I can listen to music and relax whilst I am doing the laundry

I love it when all my clothes are freshly laundered and I can wear anything I want

I save so much time finding things when all the laundry is put away

When I hang up my clothes, I save time doing the washing

When I take my clothes straight out of the washing machine and hang them up, I save time ironing

The process of setting your intention to achieve the desired result is integral to all that you do. With everything that you undertake – every chore, every telephone conversation and every business meeting – it is important to think about the message that you want to convey and what you want to take away from the experience. Why spend time beating around the bush when you know what you want?

It is not necessary to know exactly what you want for your long-term future. Your thoughts, ideas and plans will change as you experience more in life. It is important, however, to always know what you want in the current moment, because if you do not know what you want, who else will be responsible for your actions?

Consider again all the things you do during the course of a normal day. Against each activity listed that you felt a *need* rather than *desire* to achieve, write down all that you want to gain from it. Look at all the positive benefits, whether direct or indirect, you gain from each aspect of this activity and list them.

Every time you engage in this activity, shift your focus from what you need to what you want to get out of it. Time yourself on each occasion you carry out this task. Then, after one week of positive thinking and conscious awareness of your desires, review how much time this activity takes you.

Activity	Time taken
Cooking a meal	day 1 _____
	day 7 _____
Eating a meal	day 1 _____
	day 7 _____
Doing housework	day 1 _____
	day 7 _____
Working in the garden	day 1 _____
	day 7 _____
Shopping for food and household items	day 1 _____
	day 7 _____
Shopping for clothes	day 1 _____
	day 7 _____
Attending to household finances	day 1 _____
	day 7 _____
Conducting business by telephone	day 1 _____
	day 7 _____
Socialising with friends	day 1 _____
	day 7 _____
Talking with friends on the telephone	day 1 _____
	day 7 _____
Working in your current job	day 1 _____
	day 7 _____
Attending business meetings	day 1 _____
	day 7 _____
Staying on top of office paperwork	day 1 _____
	day 7 _____
Participating in sports or going to the gym	day 1 _____
	day 7 _____
Going for a hair or beauty treatment	day 1 _____
	day 7 _____

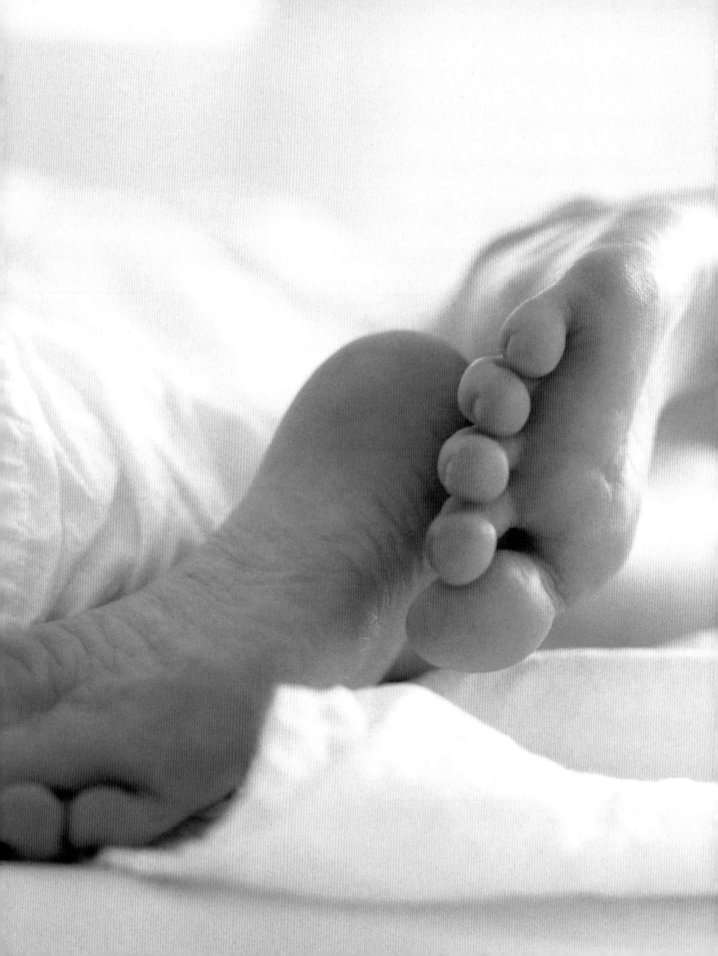

create some 'you' time

Planning your regular weekly activities is the surest way to achieve a balance of work, rest and play. Scheduling a set amount of time to get your projects done gives you a target to aim for. By thinking clearly about exactly what you want out of each experience, you are more likely to fullfil your desires in the time that you allow, as long as you have the expectation that it is achievable.

In your desire to please others, you may sometimes place yourself under unrealistic time constraints. When you are unable to meet deadlines on a consistent basis, you are not looking realistically at your current habits. The constant failure to complete tasks can eventually lead to a lowered expectations of your own abilities.

We, as individuals, are solely responsible for every action we take. How you choose to spend your time is entirely your own decision. You have the ability to change any situation you desire. The more you are able to see your achievements as a direct result of your thoughts, the more you come to expect that you will get what you want out of every part of your day.

Create a new regular weekly agenda to plan for all that you want and desire to achieve each day. Start by scheduling the time that you will give to those essentials listed, that are necessary to keep you in the best physical form. It is important that you make a conscious effort to maintain the schedule as much as possible and to look forward to each of these nurturing activities, which are integral to having a successful day.

- Getting enough sleep, required to function at your optimum level

- Eating healthy meals at the best times, required to maintain your energy level

- Making time for personal care and hygiene

- Participating in daily programmed relaxation

We all suffer time limitations based on schedules that we may or may not be able to control. When time is short, you try to make up the difference. You most often give up the things that help you to recharge and provide the reserves needed to complete other more pressing activities. In attempting to do too much, your body becomes unbalanced. Tiredness is one of the most common reasons for not functioning at your highest capacity.

For each segment of your working day that is over two hours long, plan a fifteen minute relaxation break to gain a quick fix of energy. If sleepy, start with a large glass of mineral water, add some ice, lemon or lime for inspiration, and drink with the intention that it is helping the flow of water and air throughout your body. It is also helping to hydrate your skin.

Set aside five minutes to sit quietly and practise controlled breathing; this will centre your energy. If you have nervous energy, imagine with each breath out you are exhaling your excess energy. If you are lacking in energy, imagine each breath that you draw in begins from the ground and brings with it essential earth energy to keep you connected.

30-day action plan

In order to sort your life, you must realise that you are the only one responsible for creating your reality. The decisions you make about how to look after yourself affect how you feel. You choose how you want the world to see you. You decide how you spend your time. Use this 30-day action plan to change your bad habits by taking time out to think about what you want, get excited and see what happens. You will not be disappointed.

goal	imagine	stimulate	create	appreciate	observe
Change one habit that makes you feel bad physically	**1** Think about replacing the bad habit with something good. Imagine everything that makes your body feel better on all levels. Do this when you are tempted.	**2** Walk in a relaxing space. With your feet on the ground, think about your connection to the earth. Early in the day, look at everything around you.	**3** Treat yourself today by looking after yourself. Plan to have great food, at least one hour of personal relaxation time and a good night's sleep.	**4** Do something good for your heart. Dedicate one hour today to some form of physical exercise you enjoy that will keep your heart working.	**5** Feel the difference paying attention to your physical being can make. Chart any bodily changes that have occurred over the past five days in your journal.
Improve one specific area of your appearance	**6** Think about three things to change in your life once happy with this part of your appearance. Imagine yourself as you believe you can be.	**7** Go window-shopping. Observe different people in the street. Appreciate each person's individuality, then think about your own unique qualities.	**8** Do three things today to alter your appearance. Add something, take something away and wear a different colour to change your look.	**9** Say 'thank you' whenever people compliment you on the changes you have made to your appearance. Learn to appreciate your individual style.	**10** How you feel internally is reflected in how you present yourself externally. Pay attention to how your attitude is reflected in your appearance.
Create a relaxing personal space in your home	**11** Think about creating a space, just for you, in your home. Consider the things you would include in your space and what you would do to relax.	**12** Try out any potential space to see how it feels during the time you set aside for yourself. Write down the reasons you find the space relaxing.	**13** Decide where is most relaxing. Decorate with treasured possessions. Bring anything into your space you find calming and inspirational.	**14** Take time each day to be with yourself. An hour is ideal, but even 30 minutes of solitary meditation or relaxation will help to restore your spirit.	**15** Note down how you feel after being in your space. Whenever the pressures of the day take over, recreate this space and take time out for yourself.

16 Release stagnant energy from one area of your home

Think about an area at home you no longer enjoy. Consider all items with no meaning or function. Imagine how you would rather utilise the space.

17 Spend some time in this area and open the windows. Let some air flow through the space. Make a list of ways you could improve the space.

19 Burn a scented candle in the refreshed space to clear and fragrance the air and bring new warmth into the room.

20 Pack up items no longer relevant to your lifestyle. Give them away to charity or friends, or sell them on. Open up the space to the energy of new things.

Journalise how this space feels now redundant items have been removed. Think about additional ways to make the space reflective of your current needs.

21 Change the way you feel about one task that you try to avoid

Think about the necessary skills to perform the task. Write a job description including what is expected with a great sales pitch of why the job is interesting.

22 Approach anyone who enjoys and succeeds at similar things. Ask them what they like most about what they do. Ask them the tricks of the trade.

24 Revel in the knowledge that when you want a result you can find ways to get it. Practice smiling each time you accomplish something you want.

Write down advantages of getting the job done then think of ways to enjoy the process. Focus on what you want to accomplish. Do not quit.

25 How do you feel now you accomplish something you previously found difficult? Clock how much time you save doing jobs you once avoided.

26 Use your time more efficiently in one part of your life

Imagine a video of all you did yesterday. Replay the tape looking at areas where you got things done and felt good about your accomplishments.

27 Plan to spend the spare time gained by getting into the swing of tasks. Consider incorporating uplifting elements into everything you do.

Set aside at least two hours to start and finish a project that you have been meaning to do but have never found the time to complete.

29 How does it feel to make the time to complete a task in one go? When you are on a roll, in the groove or going with the flow, it stimulates your heart.

30 Make time each day to reflect upon the elements you liked and those you did not. Look at where you put your attention and then at the end result.

goal   imagine   stimulate   create   appreciate   observe

well done Take the day to appreciate all that you have achieved in the last 30 days. See how it feels to let go of a few old ways of thinking. See how it feels.

Do something extra special today that makes you really happy and see how that feels. Give thanks to everyone that has helped you along the way to achieve your goals.

time to **reassess**

The essential skills you need to learn in order to live comfortably in the present moment are easy to master. You can improve your appearance and self-esteem, revamp your personal space and organisation skills, and alter your attitudes to daily tasks. All it takes is focus, positive energy and the belief in your own ability to see a project through to completion. But how many of these skills are becoming part of your daily life?

Become what you eat

Paying attention to your physical body is your main focus when trying to keep on the right path. When your body is well looked after, rest assured, you are doing what you know is right for you. When you neglect those things that you know you need – sufficient sleep and relaxation, nourishing food and water – your body protests and tells you something is not right.

You need daily energy that you derive from food and water, as well as from the places, people and things that surround you. In order to appreciate your physical being, you must create a routine that nourishes your existence.

Look like you feel

The way you present yourself through your dress and personal grooming reflects the importance that you give to your physical presence in various situations. When you are very comfortable and relaxed with the company you keep, you may find that you can be natural

in your appearance, in keeping with the type of occasion. Other circumstances dictate that you conform to a mode of dress. How has your appearance changed in the last thirty days? Have you taken a good look in the mirror to see whether you are revealing your inner feelings to those around you?

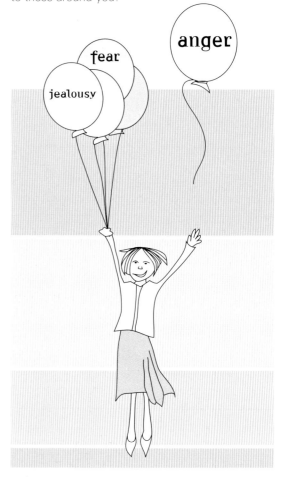

Release your emotions

It is important to let go of any anger, hatred, bitterness, sadness, disappointment or jealousy that you allow to block your path towards getting what you want. It is often far too convenient to blame others for your own unhappiness as it means you never have to confront the real issues. By writing down all that you are willing to forgive and forget, you open the pathway to receiving what you now desire.

Surround yourself with useful things

Apply this as a rule of thumb when deciding whether things have a place in your home, and indeed, your life. Any item that simply brings you pleasure also has a place in your life. Do you use it, cherish it and love it? Does it make your world a better place by being a part of it? What is it about it that makes you care so much? Do you know when to let things go?

Set your intention

Throughout your day, before you begin each task, take at least one minute to focus on what you wish to achieve. Think about all you you want to learn and what you want to teach. Set a time within which you aim to achieve this task. Do not set yourself up for constant failures. Make it a realistic goal; you must believe that you can complete it during this time.

Step forward

Paying attention to the signs that your physical body exhibits is integral to achieving a harmonious relationship with who you are. We each have personal codes that indicate when our bodies needs attention. Learning to honour these signals can prevent illness on all levels.

You are given just one physical body for your duration on this earth. In order to enjoy your body to the utmost, you must pay attention to the food you eat, the amount of exercise you take, and the relaxation you give to both your physical and

mental beings. How have your attitudes changed in the last month?

Learning to let go of all the things in your life that are no longer relevant to who you are in the present is the greatest way to raise the flow of energy throughout your body. By releasing all of the blockages in the area of your heart – all the bitterness, sadness, disappointment, anger, jealousy or hatred, it is possible to feel recharged on every level. By letting go of the physical clutter that acts as a barrier to energy flowing throughout your home, new ideas can emerge from the space, suitable for comfortable living.

Through setting your intention you can bring about change in all areas of your life. Getting through daily routines is more pleasurable when you know what you desire from each situation. By looking for what you want, you always seem to find it.

Reassess your attitudes today by looking back over the Body Consciousness and Home Comforts sections of the Positive Behaviour Survey on pages 20–3 and re-evaluating your new position. Are you feeling and looking better? Are you more comfortable in yourself and in your home? Are you managing to get more done? Have your relationships and communication skills improved?

Now review your 30-day action plan. Pick your greatest achievement out of the five goals and write down how it feels to have succeeded. Why do you think you were able to succeed? If you were writing pointers to someone on how to succeed at their goal, what advice would you give them?

Pick your greatest challenge of the five goals from the Sort Your Life 30-day Action Plan. Write down which things got in the way of making it easy to succeed. Did you lack the belief in yourself that you were able to succeed? Using the Solve Your Problems Positive Action Exercise shown on pages 90–1, use the easiest, quickest and best solutions and affirmations to overcome the challenge.

achieve your **dreams**

"If one advances confidently in the direction of his dreams,
and endeavours to live the life which he has imagined,
he will meet with a success unexpected in common hours."
Henry David Thoreau

In order to achieve your dreams, you must learn that there is a natural rhythm to life. Energy must come in and then flow out. You gain energy through your thoughts, which flow throughout everything that you create. The easiest and most fun way to encourage your creativity is to learn to stimulate your imagination and infuse everything you do with positive energy. The old saying 'seeing is believing' can be true: if you can dream something in your mind's eye there is no reason why you cannot make it a reality.

Each of us experiences our imagination differently, as the imagination includes all of our senses. By stimulating your imagination using every sensory power, the excitement generated by this stimulation propels your creative process. Most importantly, it adds fun to everything you do.

It is not enough just to use your imagination to get whatever you want. The most important thing is that you must believe that you can achieve your dreams. If you look back at your disappointments, in all probability, you did not truly believe that you would get what you wanted, which led to your failure. The power of positive thinking is an integral component of your success formula.

A good measure of how close you are to achieving your dreams is to assess how you feel. Looking at the amount of energy you are able to summons for each particular task helps you to see the areas where you may need to kick-start your system by immediately changing your attitude from negative to positive. Start to use your imagination to summon more energy for the goals that you have set for yourself.

By using the 30-day Action Plan at the end of this chapter, you can imagine an achievable goal – one that you really believe you can attain – and use the processes of stimulation, creation, observation and appreciation to achieve that goal. The very process of successfully obtaining small goals throughout the thirty days will alter your outlook forever, boost your self-esteem and allow you to believe that you can obtain your innermost desires. Remember to acknowledge all the help you gain along the way to achieving your dreams.

Sometimes in the excitement of the process, you start thinking about many things all at the same time. This can lead to confusion. In order to bring clarity to each objective, the 30-day Action Plan focuses on one goal at a time for a period of five days. The individual goals focus on the areas of your life that you wish to change.

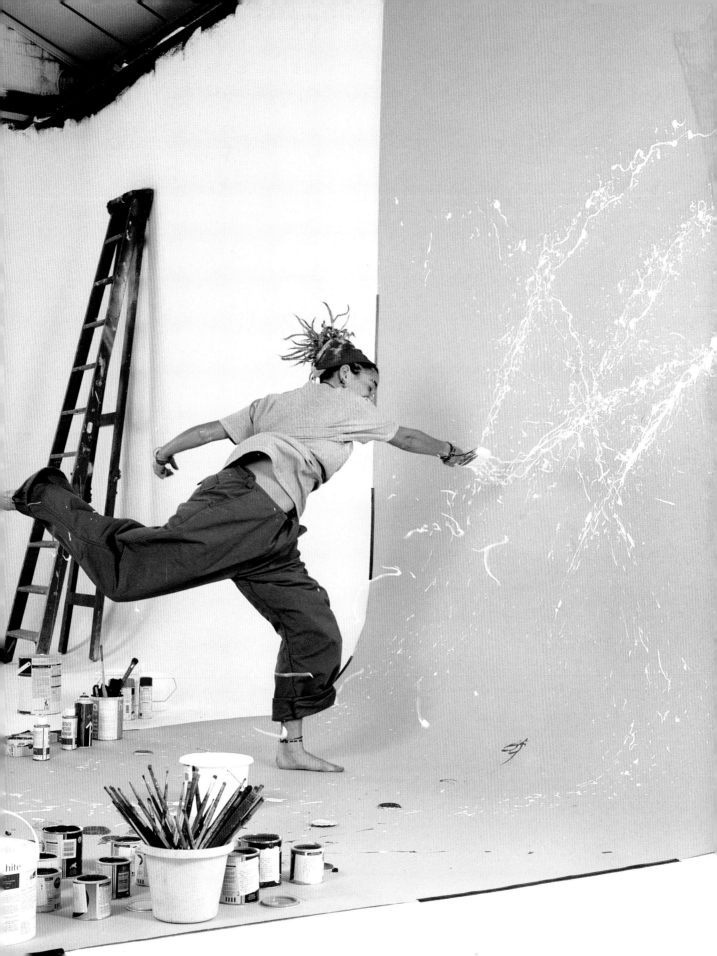

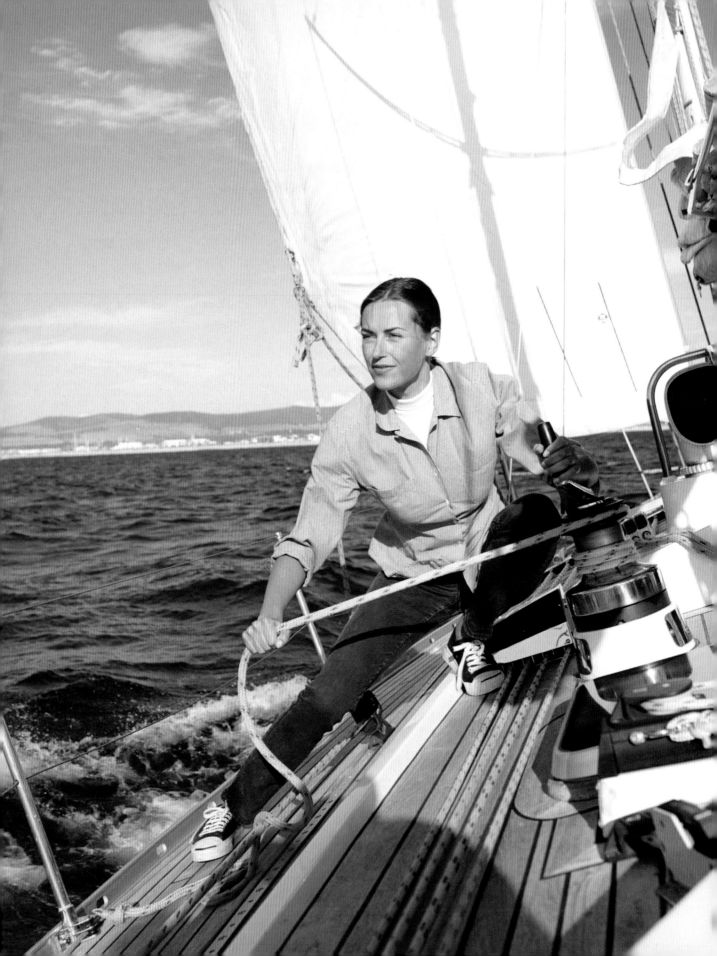

dare to dream

We all have the ability within ourselves to achieve anything we set our heart on, as long as we believe that we can achieve it. Each time you achieve something, you have directed your thoughts and emotions towards what you wanted in that moment. The power of your wanting led you to take all the necessary actions to get the object of your desire. You focussed your energy on one specific goal and made something happen.

If you look at anyone who has achieved great success in some area of their life, you will see that the underlying reason for their success was an unshakeable belief in their idea and in their ability to succeed. However, their path may not always have been smooth sailing. They could easily have been defeated along the way by listening to others who may not have believed as strongly in their ideas or abilities. Yet they chose to see those things that were positive in each situation and continued to pursue their vision until they succeeded.

You can only achieve what you dare to dream. No matter how dire your situation seems or how restrictive your circumstances, you must not let your current predicament limit your desire for something better. Getting stuck where you are is to forget that it is by the desire for something better and being proactive in pursuing it, rather than through bemoaning your current woeful lack, that you get what you want. Thinking only about what is, keeps you firmly rooted in your day-to-day reality and leaves no possibilities for transformation and change.

Thinking about something better is taking control through your thoughts and making it a reality: if you can imagine it, you can achieve it. It is only by letting go of all of the excuses for why you cannot have what you want, that you stop looking to others to make your choices for you. Become responsible for your own actions.

The best thing you can do to further your achievements is to acknowledge and feel good about each one, no matter how small it may seem at the time. The more you are able to see the power of your thoughts in action, the more you are able to build self-confidence in your abilities. It is by truly expecting that you can make things happen that you derive the motivation to go for it. If you are defeated before you begin, you will remain defeated.

Your cumulative experiences, as well as new opportunities that present themselves daily, form the basis of your dreams, which means they are ever-changing. When you were little, you may have dreamt of being a ballet dancer or a sports hero; you based those dreams on your limited experience of the world. As you develop your innate abilities, however, you may indeed go on to become a ballet dancer or sports hero, or you may go on to explore your own unique talents and make the most of them. You are able to continue to learn and accomplish new things for as long as you have the desire.

motivate yourself

The motivation to pursue your dreams comes from a wide variety of experiences, starting at an early age. As children, you are often positively motivated by rewards that your parents put in place to instil habits that they believe to be important. These positive rewards are either emotional, such as praise or affection, or material, such as money or objects. You may still be motivated by the same rewards as you progress into adulthood.

Other positive motivation can come in the form of a mentor, life coach, or any inspirational model that helps you to realise your full potential. The role of an inspirational guide is to accentuate your positive abilities and enhance them by showing the way towards gaining a greater understanding through study and concentrating your efforts towards mastering that skill. Choosing to apprentice or study under someone that you respect can put you on the path to follow in their footsteps, either teaching or utilising those skills.

Trust your instincts

When you are positively motivated, you are engaged in the process of imaging what you want and visualising the end result. The more you can employ all of your senses to stimulate your thoughts concerning that end result, the more all of your senses will point you in the direction of what you want. You become aware of things that you see, read or encounter that are relative to your thoughts and allow your sixth sense – your intuition – to help guide you in this process. You know that you are on the right track because you feel good when you make things happen.

Create some magic

Sometimes, motivation can be derived from a negative source, such as avoiding punishment, needing or lacking something or fearing failure due to past associations or future implications. Although you may be motivated to achieve your dreams out of these reasons, it is most likely that you will not enjoy the process. Feelings of desperation lead you into taking actions that are not harmonious with your real intentions. People who achieve out of need are rarely satisfied with their achievements and may feel physical symptoms indicating a lack of balance.

Sadly, there are people who have horrific experiences in their childhood that they must overcome in order to feel a worthy individual. These feelings affect your ability to reach your fullest potential. Professional help may be required in order to accept the past, and move on towards the future. Forgiving yourself and others for past experiences can take time, but is essential to your development.

The best motivation comes from within. True power comes from knowing that you have the ability to create magic and, in reality, that is exactly what you do every day. When you think about even the smallest thing and make it happen, you are seeing the results of your thoughts. Focus your attention on all you receive on a daily basis and, through gratitude, you will feel the positivity in your heart. Feeling good just cannot be beat.

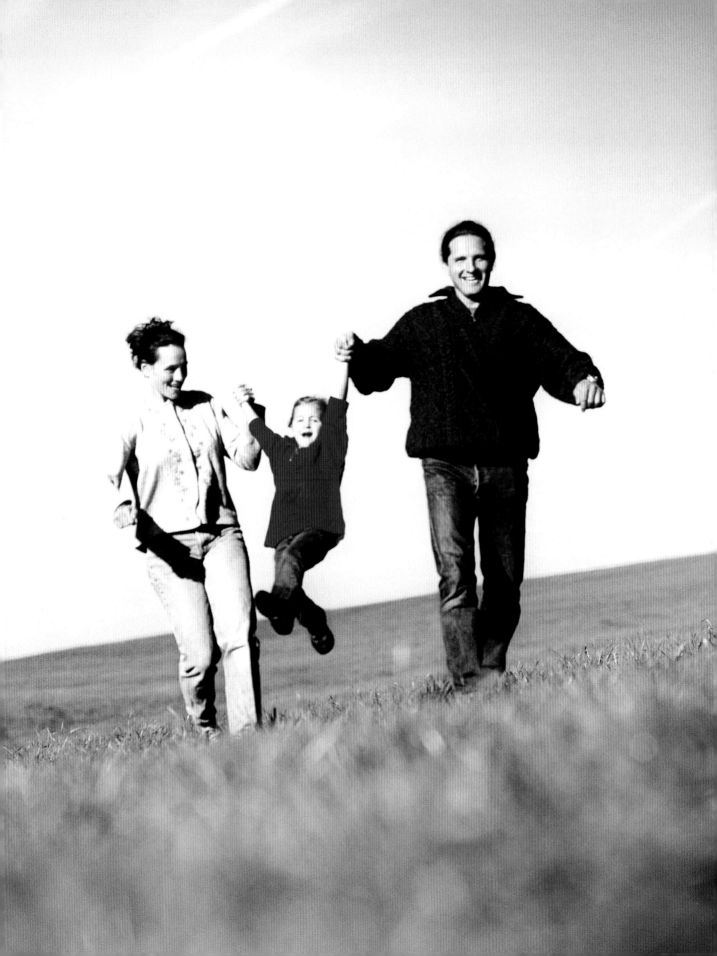

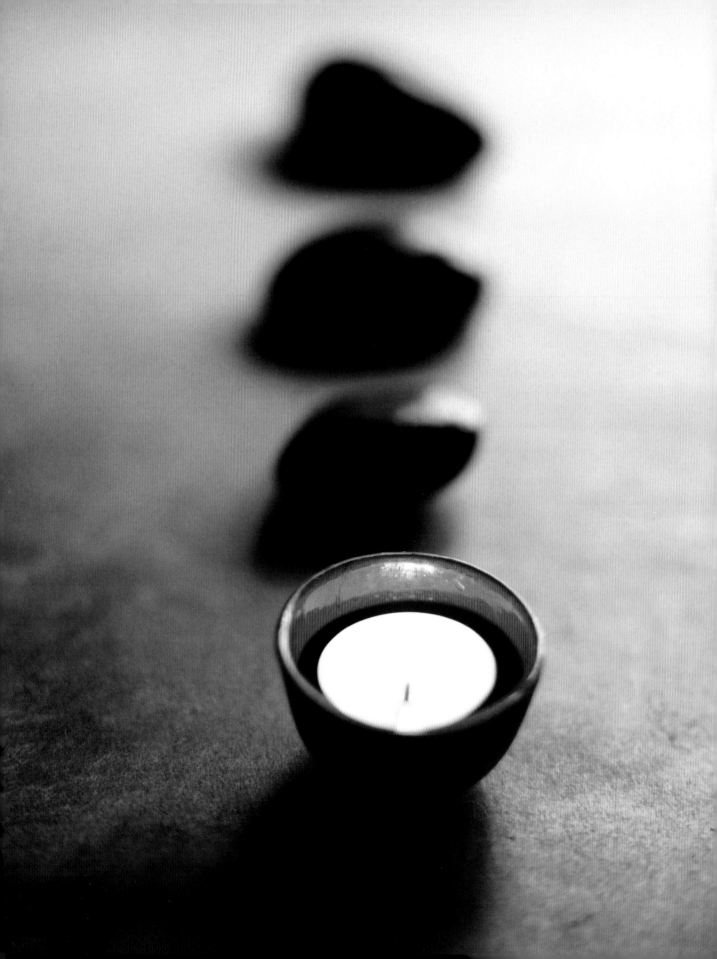

kindle the flames

Throughout the centuries, fire has been symbolic of a process of transformation and purification. When you kindle the flame of a fire, you add the necessary ingredients of fuel or air to keep it alight. Kindling your own inner flame requires not only air, food and water – life's necessities – but you also need to stoke your inner passion, which stems from your heart.

There are many ways to stoke up passion, but the most effective is dedicating time to contemplate the object of your desire. Creatively looking at ways to make things happen adds excitement to the whole process of achieving your dreams. However, creativity does not just mean artistic or visual flair. Being creative means exploring all ideas relative to what you are trying to achieve and going for those methods that make you feel good inside.

Stimulate your senses

The best way to stimulate the most ideas, is simply to think about what you want from the situation. Your imagination is your greatest tool for creative thought. When you were young, you used your imagination as a means of whiling away the hours. You created magical places, imaginary friends, and used your senses of smell, touch, hearing, taste, and vision to learn about the world. Reading is another method of stimulating your imagination, and is one of the first skills you learn as a child.

Whenever you plan for something in the future, use your imagination to think about what that upcoming event will be. Planning a holiday is a great example of using your imagination to visualise something that you will enjoy in the future. Looking at holiday brochures tantalises your senses, then your imagination fills in the blanks. The process of dreaming about something in the future actually extends the experience of the event. You feel the positive effects before, during and after. Feelings always emanate from your heart, and generally the prospect of going on a holiday makes you feel good both physically and mentally.

Extend the pleasure

To further kindle the flames of your passion, you can stimulate your imagination by physically doing something to think about it further. Going back to the holiday, you may go out and buy a book about the area you are going to visit and begin to read up on things you would like to do. You may get motivated to take some physical exercise in order to feel your best whilst you are away. Even writing down a list of things to do to prepare for the holiday stimulates your thoughts. This anticipation makes you even more excited about the future event and, in turn, stimulates your heart.

The more you think and do, the more you get out of each situation. When you look for the things that you want, you focus your energy on seeing the relevant information to help you achieve that goal. As you stimulate your thoughts by physically doing something to further challenge your mind, you stimulate your heart and feel more enthusiastic. Your focussed thoughts and stimulation, make you feel better physically and emotionally.

focus your attention

>> positive action exercise

Whatever you choose to focus your attention on, you will reap the benefit of your concentrated thoughts. Even the simplest daily tasks, such as journeying to work, can take on a whole new light when you put your energy and attention into gaining enjoyment from the experience.

In each situation you need to look at all the different experiences you want to gain from those particular circumstances. Through reading a novel, you may want to stimulate your imagination and escape into a different reality, giving your mind time to relax from your day-to-day thoughts. In the same way your intention in reading can be relaxation, you can sometimes read books to gain a specific insight on a particular topic. In this case you are not intending to relax and escape, you are seeking to engage more actively, to uncover and retain the information that you are thirsting for.

Too often, you go through your day habitually switched off from what is going on around you, and you don't think about what you want. True, things you care about get your attention, and that feels good. But, those things that you are not really bothered about, because they have become routine, often feel more like a nuisance instead of a pleasure. The things that have ceased to feel pleasurable, require you to refocus your energy on what you want right in this moment.

Pick a different activity each day, for the next week, from the list on the opposite page that you tend to neglect. Make the decision to give it your undivided, proactive attention. The first and foremost rule is to decide to enjoy the experience as your number one priority. Think about what you would like to gain from each experience.

Write down how it felt to pay special attention to one activity. Set aside 15 minutes every evening to list all the things that you enjoyed about the experience, thinking about how it made you feel on all levels – physical, mental, emotional and spiritual.

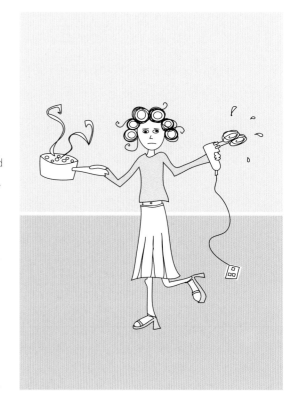

- Starting and finishing a project

- Paying bills or dealing with paperwork

- Travelling by any means of transport

- Taking a walk

- Preparing a meal

- Having a personal conversation

- Getting dressed to go out

- Playing a competitive game

- Reading the newspaper

Think about all the things you gained from this new way of approaching a old task. Compare how the experience felt when you took the helm to get what you wanted to how it usually feels when you simply go with the tide. Did you get more done?

Know what you want

We often think of our dreams as being long-term goals, or things that we will achieve by the end of our lives. As such, they often get put on the back burner to make way for more pressing issues, which we believe we need in the present. By approaching your dreams as far-off, distant maybes, you are not taking the time to create them on a daily basis and therefore are not making certain that you are leading the life you always want.

You may not feel that you have understood your true purpose in life. When those around you seem to have more direction, this, in itself, can create some anxiety. Without purpose, you drift from situation to situation, never feeling fulfilled. Sometimes, contemplating the big picture can be just too overwhelming. Because you think of so many things, you have too much stimulation of thought that leads feelings of confusion. Rather than trying to figure it all out before fitting in the pieces, it is far easier to know what you want each day.

Consider the generalities of what you want: this is sometimes easier than thinking about the specifics, especially if they are miles away from where you are in the present. You have to believe or expect that you will get what you want. Something you do not believe is obtainable, will be impossible to reach. For example, if you weigh 25 stone but want to be 10 stone, if you believe your expectation is unrealistic, losing 15 stone can prove an immense challenge. If, however, you dream of losing two pounds each week you are focussed on the single issue of controlling your weight for the day, rather than thinking about all the ways you will have to control your weight over the many months it will take to achieve the end result. Which feels better? The small achievement of the day or the worry about whether you will ever get to the end?

Enjoy the daily experiences: this is the best way to make the most out of each situation. Everyone says the journey is the bit that counts. You never know when the journey is going to end, so focussing on getting what you want from each situation will enable you to feel good each day and never regret what you could have done. You need to explore the many methods that you can employ to feel good each day and actively pursue them. Each minute of the day can be made happier and more efficient by consciously choosing to enjoy the experience. From the moment you awake, you can look for inspiration, laughter, guidance, relaxation or stimulation. You can go out into the world and look around to view the contrasts and the similarities, and through this process gain a greater understanding of what you want.

Stay in touch with your daily dreams. Be aware of all that you achieve each day. Taking time to acknowledge your accomplishments, shows that you have noticed the results of your thoughts and actions, and have learned from the experience. Every small step forward is a step in the right direction.

seeing is believing

Once you are able to focus your attention and see the results of your actions, you will be able to gain belief in your own abilities. Expectation, belief and faith are all words for the deeper understanding that you gain when you acknowledge your own creations.

A major part of your belief structure stems from how you feel you fit into the larger scheme of the universe. Across the globe, many people seek guidance and comfort through their religious beliefs. Many practise their beliefs as a group, and from this experience also gain the emotions of the 'collective consciousness', or the feelings of the group.

This type of expectation, belief or faith can have tremendous power. Most of us have studied religious or cultural beliefs and have heard stories of spiritual healings that occurred through a faith passed down over thousands of years. Such healings still occur each day. The human mind is a powerful force. When it is combined with positive emotions, such as joy, reverence and deep-rooted belief, miracles can and do happen.

Some people may not practise an organised religion, but have their own set of values and beliefs about the cosmic questions that we all have concerning life and death. Others still may not question their role in the universe at all. Faith does not need to be attributed to any religion. Faith can simply be a belief in the law of cause and effect: if you do good things, live your life with joy and show gratitude, you will achieve your heart's desire.

Faith is belief that does not rest on logical proof or material evidence, but rather on a deeper, knowing level. When you rely on your inner-guidance system to point you in the direction of your innermost desires, you learn to have 'faith', or a deeper knowing, that there is a cause and effect to your actions. The more profoundly you understand that how you think, feel and expect things to happen affect how things do actually turn out, the greater control you'll have over your destiny.

Believe in yourself

Once you learn how to do something, you can repeat it whenever you desire. You come to expect, believe or have faith that you can do it. Learning to trust your own abilities is the only thing between you and your dreams. Think about the first time you ever rode a two-wheeled bicycle on your own. Remember how it felt to learn something new and with the knowledge that you can do it again and again.

You learn things by repetition: when you incorporate something into your basic store of knowledge, you keep it with you forever. To remember an experience, you must make it memorable. When you perform a ritual to commemorate an experience, as we all do in every stage of our lives, you remember the experience with emotion from your heart. Each day, it is important to commemorate the things that make you happy, as well as everything that you have received by actively thinking about what you want. Experience and remember it: you need to do something, no matter how small, to acknowledge each goal you achieve.

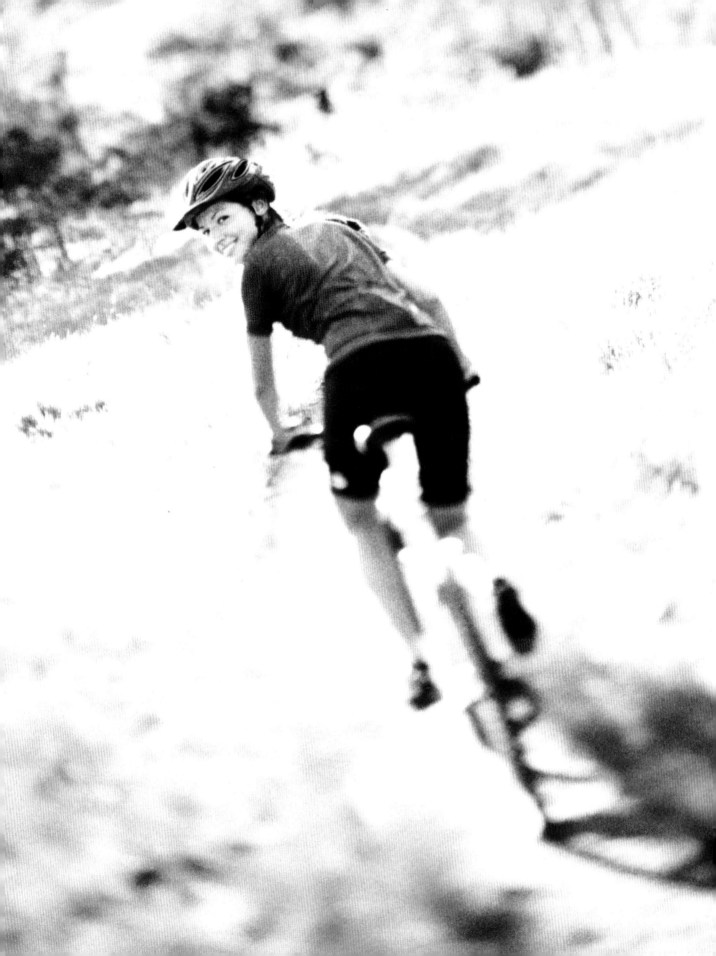

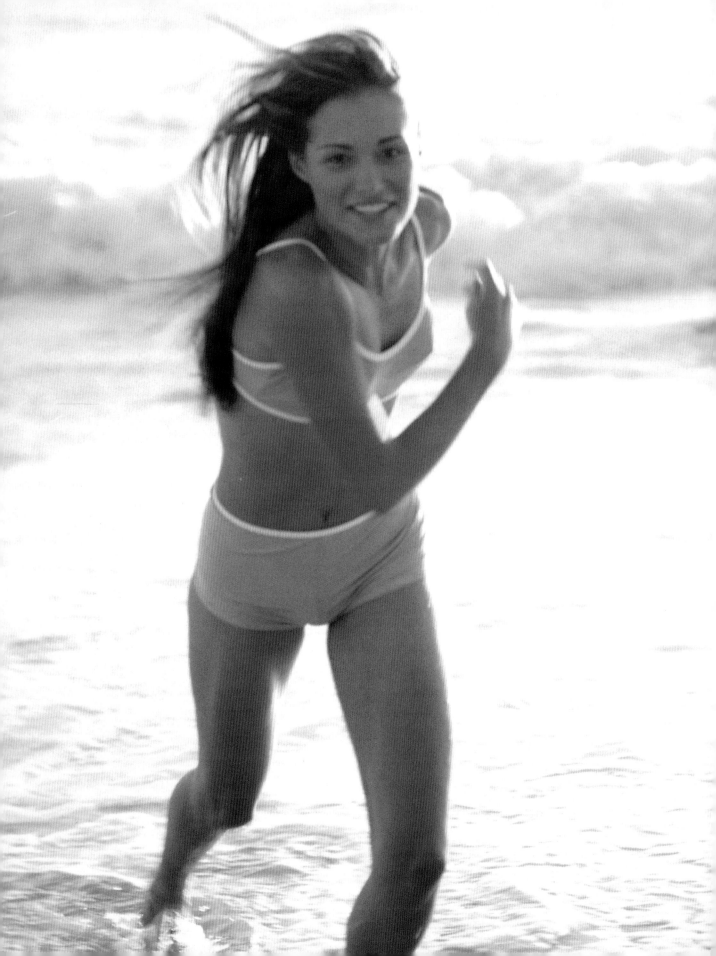

maximise your energy

On contemplating energy, you generally think about the amount of stamina that you have to get you through the day. In physical terms, you derive your energy through the food you eat, the water you drink and the air you breathe – the three elements required to maintain your life-force energy. Likewise, physical exercise and relaxation are integral to keeping your body working at peak efficiency and enable you to convert food and oxygen to keep your body healthy.

You are probably able to detect your energy levels upon getting up in the morning. How you feel is often a direct result of how well you looked after yourself the day before. What you ate, whether you incorporated any relaxation into your schedule and how much sleep you had that night, directly effects the amount of get-up-and-go you have to face the day. Tiredness and physical aches and pains are often easy to remedy by going back to basics: drink sufficient water and replenish your body with food.

Understand earth's vibrations

There are, however, many other things that effect your energy on a daily basis. If you consider the broader category of energy – as all matter having a unique vibration – you realise that all types of matter can have an impact on your energetic being, and can add to or take away from your own feeling of energy.

Einstein developed the theory that all matter vibrates, and it is the frequency of the vibration that allows you to see things in their unique way. Things that you can see with the physical eye are lower in frequency than those things you cannot see, but they still exist in another form. Think about your ability to hear music. Music is a high frequency vibration that we are unable to see but are able to hear. Similarly your thoughts and emotions are vibrations, like music, of a higher frequency.

Balance your energy levels

In order to maintain a balance, you need a link with the low-frequency energies that physically connect you to the earth, as well as some of the high-frequency energies, which effect the mental, emotional and spiritual levels of your being. Getting to grips with how to regulate the energy you require when you need it, is a skill that can be learned.

We can all feel a little 'spacey' after spending too much time in our thoughts. If you are lost in your own head, connected to high-frequency energies, you lack a connection to what is going on around you. In essence, you are not grounded. Creative types may suffer from a lack of grounding. No earth connection can become physically manifest in a weakened immune system. Illnesses such as ME, eczema, and poor circulation may benefit from consciously seeking low-frequency energies.

Likewise, if you have too much low-frequency energy, you are deeply rooted to your beliefs and cannot see the greater picture. You find it difficult to use your imagination as you have lost your connection to the high-level frequencies. This prevents you from embracing your beliefs and feelings. Having too much low-frequency energy blocks any energy you may receive from sources you cannot see.

harness the earth's energies

We have all experienced moments of awareness when it is become apparent how our energy is affected by the environments we find ourselves in and the situations we choose to participate in. By way of example, you may find that you gain energy when you are out in the sunshine or digging in the garden.

You may find that some people seem to give you energy and you feel enthused after you have spent time with them. Conversely, other people seem to drain your energy and take without giving anything back. You may also find that some material or natural objects give you energy, such as crystals, works of art or the wonders of nature. You may even be aware that certain colours, scents or music can give a boost to your energy levels.

Keep your energy flowing

By understanding the different types of energy that you require to achieve balance, you can regulate your energy. The founding principle of all energy-healing techniques is to call upon the earth's energies to establish a balance, release blockages and allow the energy to flow throughout the body. Even without studying specific energy-healing techniques, you can learn to recognise the signs that your body gives off according to the type of energy that you require daily. Paying attention to the physical and emotional signals that you need balance enables you to use various techniques to achieve the energy you require for any occasion.

Assess your electromagnetism

We are all electromagnetic beings with most of us falling somewhere in the middle of the electro-magnetic spectrum. Some of us, however, sit at either end of the scale, being either highly magnetic or highly electric. Those on the magnetic end of the spectrum tend to attract other people's energies. This means that they can walk into a crowded room and feel the other people's illnesses or problems. This can be overwhelming and distressing, but can be dealt with, to some extent, through the healing techniques discussed on pages 84–5.

One sign that you may be highly magnetic is if you have problems keeping watches working properly, whereas those on the electric end of the spectrum can have problems with electricity. I am a highly-electric person, so when my energy is unbalanced, I can burn out several lightbulbs in a single day, simply by turning on a switch.

Highly electric people can have problems with computers and other electronic equipment. Simple grounding exercises, such as those explained on pages 84–5, can help discharge excess energy and should be practiced as a matter of routine to keep your energy from becoming too electric. No one enjoys getting or giving shocks on a daily basis.

You have the power to utilise the earth's energies to maximise your potential and allow your magnificent human body to work at its most efficient level. All it takes is the clarity of your thoughts to summon up what you need in each moment.

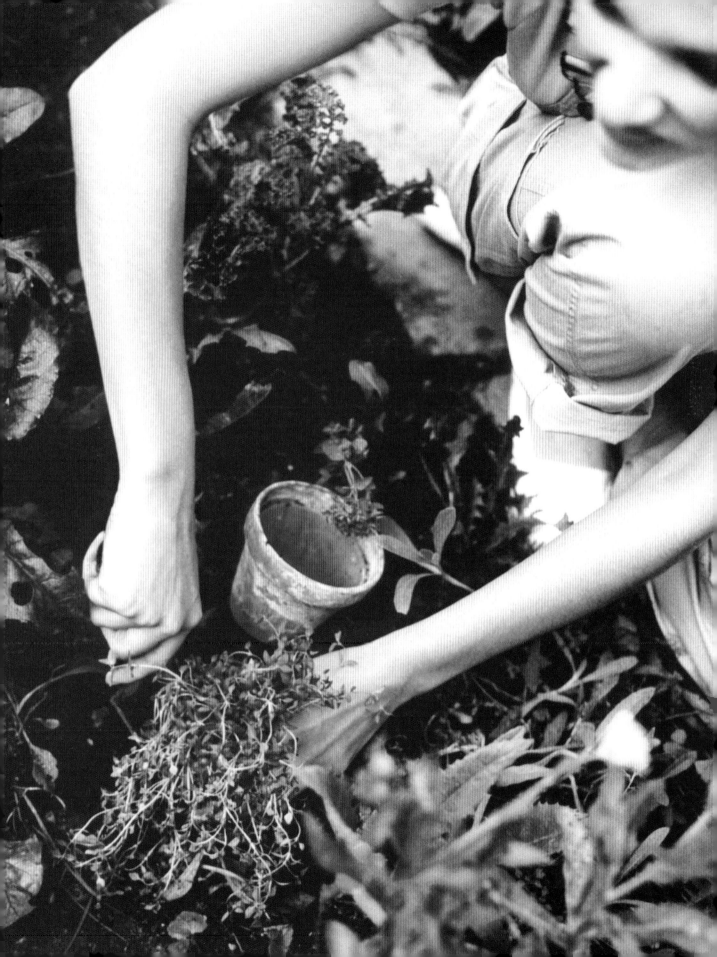

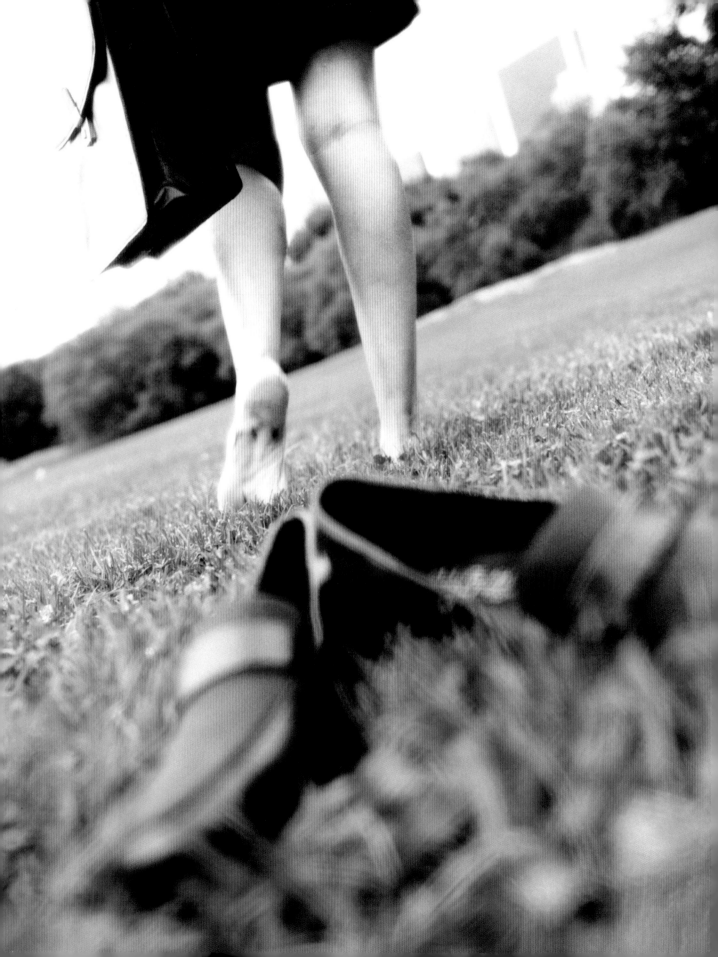

take a walk on the wild side
>> positive action exercise

Most of us experience a lack of energy at some point during the day, which can usually be resolved by eating well or having a good night's sleep. But when you find your energy is low on a consistent basis, with no physical causes, it can mean that you are spending too much time in your own head and not enough time connected to the earth and those things that are going on around you.

There are many ways to get a quick boost of earth energy. The easiest is to do something that physically connects you with the earth. Try the following quick-fix methods to feel the earth's energy, clear your mind and give you physical stamina.

Plug into the earth's energy

Connect with the natural elements by going for a walk in your favourite outdoor space. This can be as close to home as your own garden or you can take a special trip to your favourite park or beach.

Take off your shoes and socks, and, if the weather permits, go for a long walk barefooted so you can directly feel the earth or sand under your feet. Feel the coolness of the energy in your feet as they are rooted to the earth. If you are unable to remove your shoes for the walk, simply know that the amazing earth energy is connecting to your body through your feet.

Imagine the earth's energy is replenishing your batteries, as you are walking. Become aware of your breathing. Take a deep breathe in,

breathing through your diaphragm, keeping your shoulders in place. As you breathe in, feel the earth energy begin to enter through the soles of your feet and gradually start to rise up to your ankles. Become aware of the feeling of warmth in your ankles, as the energy begins to rise up your legs to your knees. Become aware of your knees and feel the warmth start to circulate up your legs as is starts to travel to your hips.

Continue to take good deep breaths as the energy travels up your spine through your solar plexus, your heart, your throat and up through the crown of your head. As you feel the energy circulating throughout your body, you begin to feel stronger and more connected to the earth. Your batteries are beginning to become fully charged, and you are able to feel a connection with all of the natural elements around you.

Pay attention to the beauty all around you. You are part of the universe and physically connected to the earth. As you complete your walk, you feel energised and can think clearly. You feel one with the earth and understand that you can plug into to this source of energy anytime you feel depleted.

Any time you need any energy boost, think back to this time you have spent physically connecting with earth and recreate the experience in your mind to recapture the feelings of this essential life-force energy.

regulate your energy

Sometimes you can have too many thoughts and ideas bouncing around inside your head, which makes you feel like you have too much energy. This can make you nervous and on edge. Excess energy also makes it difficult to feel physically connected to the earth, leading to problems in getting things done.

Living inside your head can lead to confusion. Learning to quiet your mind and channel your excess energy through a variety of methods can dramatically reduce stress and improve your ability to see things through to completion.

You can use any of these methods to release your excess energy and give your mind a break. Like anything, practice makes perfect. At the beginning, if your mind starts to wander, do not worry. Gently bring your attention back to the exercise.

Dig your cares away

One of the easiest and fastest methods of alleviating excess energy is to get digging. Gardening helps to relax your mind and channel surplus energy into the earth. This Postive Action Exercise is a simple way to feel the benefits of more balanced energy levels.

Work the soil with your hands for at least twenty minutes. As explained on page 79, your thoughts and emotions are comprised of higher-frequency energies. In order to achieve an equilibrium, you must release unwanted thoughts and worries into the ground.

Close your eyes and take deep breaths, as deep as you can, as you begin to dig in your garden.

Remember to keep your shoulders relaxed when you breathe: avoid building tension rather than relieving it.

Bury your hands in the soil, with your eyes still closed, and take a few minutes to feel the coolness of the earth against your skin. Feel the lower-frequency earth energy.

You may feel a tingling sensation coming up through your hands. Imagine it travelling across your body. Feel your feet firmly connected to the ground.

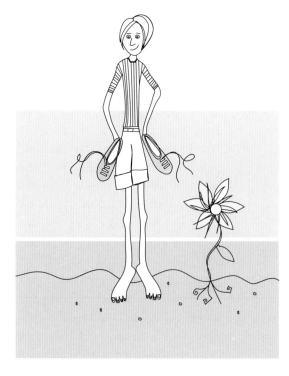

Slowly open your eyes and envisage all of your unnecessary thoughts and worries travelling from the top of your head, down through your brow, across your heart and then out through the palms of your hands into the earth. You may feel an electric tingle, as the excess energy begins to pour into the earth.

Even if you do not have a garden, you can still do this exercise by filling a plant pot with soil and placing your hands in the potted earth. Sit in a chair with your feet firmly on the ground, holding the plant pot in your lap.

Ground yourself through meditation

This grounding mediation can be done at any time of the day. Set aside twenty minutes of uninterrupted time and, if possible, sit in an upright chair and wear loose and comfortable clothing to feel entirely at ease.

Sit with your feet on the ground and your spine pressed up against the back of the chair. Close your eyes and take three deep breaths, breathing through your diaphragm but keeping your shoulders still.

Focus your attention on your feet and feel their connection to the earth. Imagine that you are a tree with your deep root structure reaching far down into the soil. Envisage the type of tree that you are and feel your root system spreading deep into the ground.

Continue with your controlled breathing. On each breath out, imagine all of your unwanted thoughts and worries are travelling from the top of your head, down through your brow, across your heart, down your spine and legs and then out into the earth to be cleansed and recycled.

Feel your tension being released as it starts to dissipate into the ground. Begin to feel your neck and shoulders relax, and the pressure leaving your solar plexus, back, hips and knees. As you begin to feel stronger and more balanced, wriggle your toes,

still feeling their connection to the earth. Slowly bring yourself back into the present moment and open your eyes, maintaining your appreciation of the earth's healing energies.

Engage in physical exercise

If you cannot remain still long enough to garden or meditate, a more active way to release excess energy is to burn it off through physical exertion. Getting involved in physical exercise is a great way to disengage your mind from your day-to-day worries and alleviate surplus energy with the added benefit of improving your health and appearance. Develop a special de-stressing routine that is gentle, rather than aggressive, and take things at a relaxing, rather than competitive, rate.

Go for a swim. Spending time in the water is a great way to shed nervous energy. Set your intention to swim twenty lengths in the pool and concentrate on your breathing. Water conducts sound and energy, so listen to the rhythm of your breathing. Be aware of the physical sensation as your hand enters the water. If miscellaneous thoughts enter your mind, let them go and return to them after your swim is completed.

If you are unable to get to a pool, try the next best thing and take a hot soak in the tub. Add essential oils such as basil, bergamot, jasmine, lavender or neroli to soothe and relax an overanxious mind.

Ride a bike. Exercising in the open air heightens your senses and your awareness. You must pay attention to the things going on around you for your own safety. When you ride outdoors you connect to the natural elements and gain a sense of grounding.

Take an early morning ride in an open green space and pay attention to the natural elements. Notice the trees and plants, sky and wildlife. Feel the air as you move across the landscape. Feel your physical connection to the sun, earth and air.

dream a little dream

Each and every day, you must concentrate your energy on what you want from life. The more passionate and enthusiastic you are about your desires, the greater chance you have of achieving them. Your imagination is the most powerful tool that you have to propel you towards achieving not only your daily goals, but also your ever-changing long-term aims. In other words, your imagination helps you to create your reality.

There are two parts to the human brain – the right and left hemispheres. The left hemisphere of the brain is the centre of logic, whereas the right hemisphere of the brain houses creativity. Right-handed people mainly utilise the left side of their brain, whilst those that are left-handed are more right-brain orientated. In all cases, however, when you are in a sleeping, dream state, the right side of your brain is more active. Your conscious mind – the one anchored in the real world – is able to switch off and your unconscious mind – or your higher self – is able to communicate with you through the dream process. You can gain great insight into your feelings towards your daily life by studying the symbolic imagery in your dreams.

Engage your imagination

Whilst in a dream state, you are often trying to resolve problems or obstacles that you have created in your waking life. Your unconscious mind holds all of the positive and negative life experiences that you have accumulated over time. Your self-image, which is based on these experiences, is often expressed through your dreams. By actively engaging your right-brain imagination, you can alter your self-image and consciously change any deep held beliefs about your own self worth.

Using your imagination, or daydreaming, during waking hours activates the right side of your brain. It takes your focus off the reality of what is and utilises your creative processes to help you to see all that can be. When you engage your imagination, you are able to use all your senses to create a vision of you are thinking about. You are able to see things clearly, in perfect detail, and even to experience the smells, tastes and sounds of what you are imagining. You are able to look at things in a new light, and through this creative process, make them happen.

There are many situations in life that may benefit from imagining more creative solutions. If, for example, you have fears that inhibit you from performing certain tasks, the process of creative visualisation can enable you to experience the task as you would like to, and feel the experience of overcoming your fear and succeeding at the task. The process of creating positive feelings about the experience, even only in your imagination, can build confidence and enable you to progress to achieving your goals.

As I have already mentioned on page 76, you learn by repetition. As a child, you learnt your multiplication tables by performing them over and over again. Once you have created the vision of how you would like things to be, making time on a daily basis to re-create this vision will give you the necessary belief to make it happen.

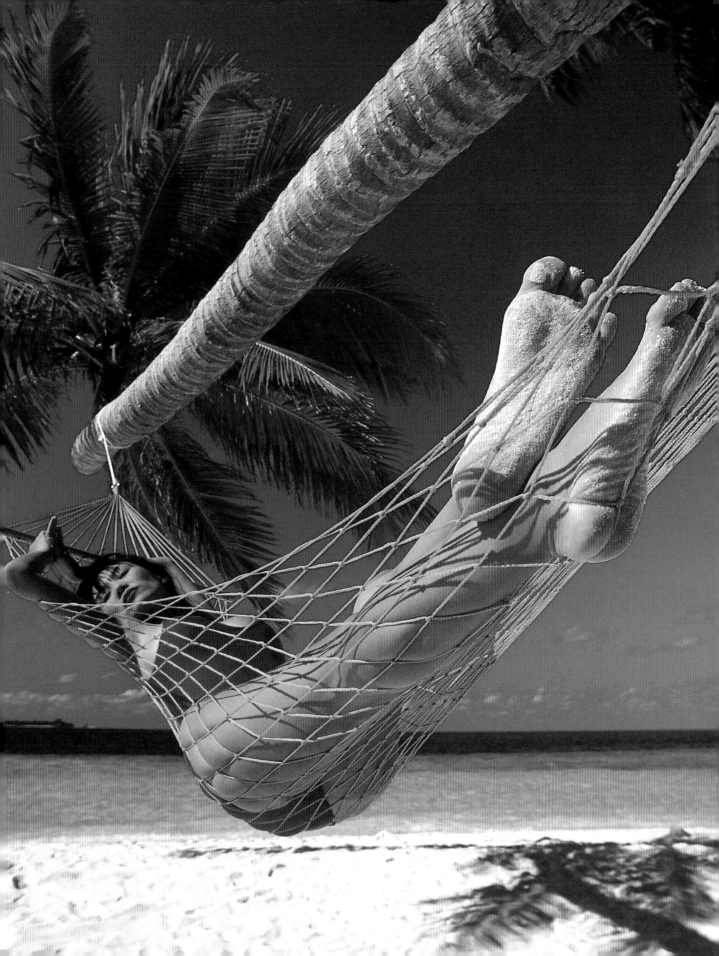

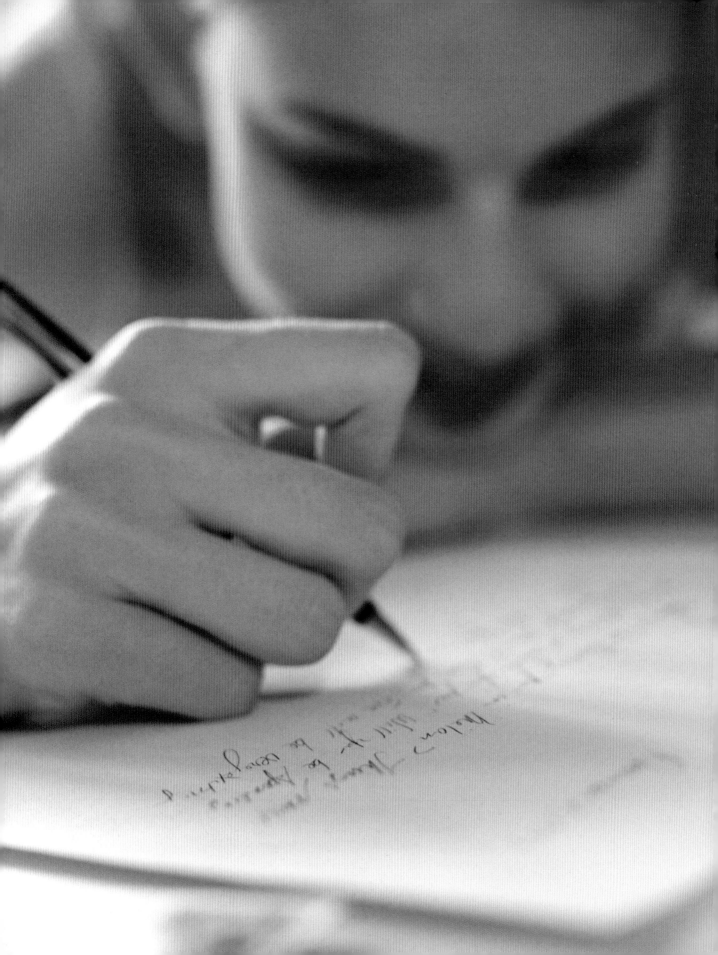

unleash your creativity

Engaging the right side of your brain helps to unleash your creative power, which comes from within and allows you to listen to your inner voice. Your inner voice is the central core of your being, the part of you that really knows what you believe and want for yourselves. When you live by your true beliefs, you will always find the path towards your dreams. At the specific points in your life when you are experiencing difficulty, it is often because you are not being true to yourself.

Your inner voice can sometimes become blocked by your conscious mind. Based on past circumstances, your logical brain encourages you to expect things to happen in a predictable way. When you are using your logical brain, you look for the sensible options that you have relied on in the past. You may hold onto these old ideas and expectations too tightly, however, and find that you are blocked in knowing what you truly want. You may be unwilling to listen to what is deep down inside your heart.

Exercise your mind

You need to exercise your creative mind to establish your connection to the higher wisdom, to gain insight into new ways to approach situations. As you come to believe that your insight, or creativity, will bring forth solutions that work, you begin to follow your intuition to help guide you on your path. Ignite the spark of creativity in your mind and it will add sparkle to everything you do.

Put pen to paper

The process of committing pen to paper forces you to think and allows you to tap into your creative resources. With the endless possibilities of a blank sheet of paper, you can create anything you want. Writing creatively does not mean sitting down and conjuring up perfect prose fit to win the Pulitzer or Booker Prize, it means looking creatively at any situation and writing about all the possible ways of working it out.

Try this exercise first thing on a morning when you do not have to go to work. Pour yourself a large cup of coffee or tea, and relax. Think about something that you want and expect to achieve in the next thirty days. It could be simply finishing the household paperwork, getting away for a weekend with your partner or a more complex task, such as finishing up a project or business proposal.

Now, put on your creative hat. Write a story at least three pages long, detailing your observations of someone else completing the same task. See how inventive you can be. Write about a completely fictious character or someone real that you do not know, a film star perhaps, doing something you are planning to do. Do not worry about your spelling or grammar, just think creatively about the situation.

Use this exercise to find new ways of doing old things. Sometimes you are more able to see things in others, rather than in yourself. What did your inner voice have to say about the situation? Did it herald any surprises?

solve your problems

We all possess creative abilities, whether we are naturally right- or left-handed, but in order to achieve balance, you need to integrate both your logical and creative beings. Your logical brain can help you to remember what you have learnt whilst your creative brain can help you to see what your next experience will be. When both logic and creativity are in harmony, you can experience both sides of the spectrum and benefit from looking at problems from each angle.

To begin with, use the problem-solving strategy that most suits the type of person you are. If you are naturally a logical person, start with the strategy for left-brain thinkers. If you are a creative person, try the method for right-brain thinkers first. In both cases, set aside an hour of personal time when you will not be interrupted. Find the most comfortable area of your home, relax and give this exercise your undivided attention.

Think creatively

This is a problem-solving strategy for right-brain thinkers, or creative types. You will need to find a comfortable chair where you can sit with your feet on the ground and your spine against the chair back.

Imagine a beautiful golden flower with many petals in front of you. You may be able to visualise it clearly, see it through a mist or perhaps just sense that it is there. Next, try to see your problem in the middle of the flower, almost as if you are watching it on a television screen.

Allow a solution to float through the screen and land on one of the beautiful golden petals. Throughout this process, you must remain neutral: do not judge whether the solution is good or bad.

Keep imaging the floating solutions coming through the problem and landing on one of the beautiful golden petals. Continue this visualisation until you have filled as many petals with solutions as you can. Now write down all of the solutions.

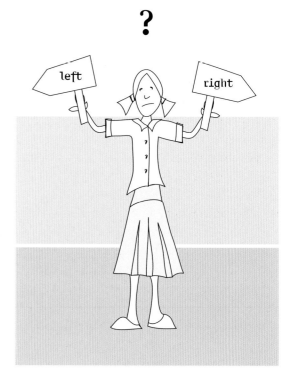

Think strategically

This is a problem-solving strategy for left-brain thinkers, or logical types. Again, you need to find a quiet corner and make yourself comfortable.

Write down a problem you want to solve on a clean sheet of paper. Jot down the first three solutions that immediately spring to mind. Do not judge whether they are good or bad solutions; write them down without questioning their merits. Now, try to think of four more solutions to the problem. Again, do not worry about how they sound, just write them down.

Think of a further eight resolutions to the problem. You may consider how a family member, friend or acquaintance would approach a similar situation. However you approach it, expand your mind into thinking about additional ways to tackle the problem. Continue this exercise until you are unable to come up with any additional solutions to the problem in question.

Prioritise your solutions

Whichever problem-solving strategy you employed, whether right- or left-brain, go back through everything you wrote down. Look for the solution that stands out as the easiest, quickest and best way to resolve your problem. Trust your instincts: if it is an easy action to take and you believe that you can do it, your inner judgement will tell you that this is the best way forward.

Mark the solution that feels best with the number '1'. Continue working through all your proposed solutions, marking the next best with the number '2', and so on until you have numbered all of the possible answers to your problem.

Write down three positive affirmations for your favoured solution. These affirmations should be positive statements of belief or intent that you will

use on a daily basis to remind you of what you want. Write each affirmation on a separate sheet of paper. For example, if the favoured solution to your problem is to write a report in three days, you may want to make the following positive affirmations.

> I enjoy thinking about my ideas as the words flow from my hand onto the page

> I can express my thoughts very clearly through my writing

> It is wonderful that my voice is heard through the reports I write

Each affirmation must be phrased in a positive way, in the present tense, and be specific to the solution. Next to each affirmation, write the date that you want the solution to be in place.

Place the sheet of paper with your first affirmation written on somewhere you are likely to see it often throughout the day. Every time you see the sheet of paper, if possible, say your affirmation out loud. If that is impractical, or just plain embarrassing, repeat the affirmation silently to yourself. Do try to pick a location that will allow you to say your affirmation out loud. Say it with feeling!

Place the two further written affirmations in other locations that you frequent daily, and get into the habit of repeating them both at least three times each day. Stating your positive belief that you are already achieving what you want, programs your conscious mind to feel the results of your thoughts. If you think that you are a creative and talented individual, you will use your inner talents to their highest and greatest good.

Chart your progress up until the date marked on your positive affirmations arrives. Continue down your list of solutions, creating positive affirmations for each solution, until you have resolved the problem.

heighten your senses

>> positive action exercise

Being creative takes practice. Although some people may be naturally gifted in expressing their creativity through music, dance, art, writing or other crafts, it is only through practice that it becomes a way of life. The more you use all of your senses, including the development of your sixth sense, or intuition, the more you will be able to fully enjoy each experience. Whilst travelling, one of my greatest delights was learning that in Bali there is no word for 'art'. Creativity is not considered a specialist skill or activity but is something that is practised each day!

Using your senses of vision, smell, taste, hearing and feeling, you possess the ability to create in your mind's eye anything that you dare to dream of. You can envisage places you have never visited through looking at a photograph. You can tangibly recall a smell in your imagination even though it is not actually present. And although you may never have seen a zebra in person, you can imagine what it would be like to pat one and feel the texture of its fur. You can probably even taste your favourite food or drink, if you try hard enough.

Creative visualisation toolkit

There are many ways of using your ability to creatively visualise and experience things through your mind's eye. For each idea listed, come up with your own creative visualisation that uses all of your senses to capture the feeling. Recall a memorable experience in your mind or create the ideal vision of what you want. Think in colour. Let your imagination go wild and take in all the details.

Motivation

Escape

Happiness

Love

Enthusiasm

Rest

Play

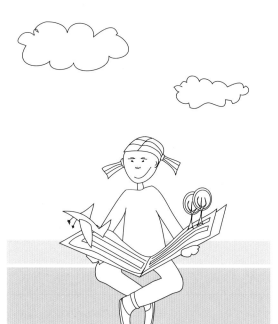

Focus on one visualisation per day, whichever feels most appropriate in that moment. Write down anything and everything that comes to mind as a result of stimulating your creative side. Use them whenever you need to feel these emotions.

Develop your intuition

There are many methods to develop your intuition. Start by becoming aware of each of your five senses, which will allow you to be more in tune with your inner wisdom. Try this exercise over the next five days and write down your experiences each day.

Become aware of your sense of sight. During the course of day one, pay great attention to the details of all that you see. Look at each area as if you are viewing it for the first time.

| Describe your house

| Describe what you are wearing

| Describe your place of work

| Describe three people you meet in your day

| Describe what you noticed in nature

You see things you have never noticed before when you decide really to observe your surroundings. Pay attention to whatever stands out as this is your inner wisdom giving guidance. By developing your outer vision, you activate your inner vision.

Activate your sense of smell and open the flow of energy. Become aware of the various scents you encounter throughout day two. List your favourite smells and why you like them. It may be the aroma of bread baking, the seaside or your favourite fragrance. Think about smells that you associate with people. Have you ever felt someone's presence in a room because of their signature fragrance? Think about fragrances that uplift or relax, and incorporate them into your routine.

Show an appreciation for the taste of all foods. All too often, we eat a meal without really tasting our food. It is easy to slip into a routine of always eating the same things. It is time to venture into new territories. During day three, list your ten favourite flavours. Describe what it is about the taste that makes your mouth water. Make the efffort to try three new items of food. Describe their taste.

Hone your sense of hearing. Selectively tune out those things that you do not wish to hear and concentrate on what you find of interest. Despite the hustle and bustle of daily life, we are able to carry on a conversation in a busy place, yet the sound of a drop of water can keep us awake. During day four, sit for fifteen minutes in a busy public place. For half of the time, listen to all the noise generated by everything around you. For the second half, focus on the sounds of just one event going on around you. Learning to focus your sense of hearing will enable you to tune in and tune out whenever you need to.

Bring awareness to the sensivity of your touch. Your hands transmit and receive energy, so you will be able to direct your energy through your sense of touch. Have you ever felt an electric shock when you touched someone that you were attracted to? Or, felt magnetically drawn towards an object? During day five, make it a point to focus on the feelings in your hands whenever you engage in any of the following. Write down all of the feelings you experience.

| Hug someone you love

| Stroke a pet

| Touch a plant

| Lay your hands on a computer, television or radio

You may experience a tingling, a sense of heat or energy, electricity or a wave of emotion. Develop this skills by staying aware of your sense of touch.

30-day action plan

In order to achieve your dreams, you must truly expect to get what you want from life. If you look back at your past disappointments, in all probability, you did not believe you would achieve a positive outcome. By using the 30-day Action Plan, you can imagine an achievable goal, one that you really believe you can attain, and use the processes of imagination, stimulation, creation, appreciation and observation to get the desired result.

goal	imagine	stimulate	create	appreciate	observe
to change a negative attitude about a situation	**1** Consider one thing you do daily that makes you feel bad. Imagine that situation with no obstacles. Think about how good this feels throughout the day.	**2** Note all the positive knock-on effects this has on your life. List the things you could further achieve by turning this negative situation into a positive.	**3** Take positive action by implementing the first achievement on your list.	**4** Give thanks to someone who helped you to achieve this action.	**5** Write down how you feel physically and emotionally when you think about this goal. Once you shift your energy relative to a subject, it is changed forever.
to change a negative attitude about a person	**6** Think about someone you know who makes you feel bad. Imagine seeing only the positive in this person and having a harmonious relationship.	**7** Note the ways this person positively contributes to any aspect of your life. Even the smallest positive contribution will change your attitude.	**8** Look for an opportunity to share a positive moment with this person.	**9** Reinforce all the ways this person has a positive impact on your life by letting them know each time you feel positive around them.	**10** Write down all the ways you feel better about yourself when you are less critical of others. Note all the changes you feel towards this person.
to regulate physical energy	**11** Think of a daily task that drains you of energy. Imagine a bank from which you can draw unlimited energy to effortlessly complete this activity.	**12** Excitement breeds energy. To up excitement levels, list everything you can do with your spare time and energy once you have completed this task.	**13** Before doing this task today, take action by getting happy before beginning. Create a fun environment in which to complete this task.	**14** Feel the physical benefit in the area around your head that increased enthusiasm generates.	**15** Note how much time this task took to complete today. Write about how you physically felt once the task was complete.

goal	to regulate mental energy	to develop short-term goals	to develop long-term strategies

16 Think about a task wher your mind often wanders. Imagine this is the only task that you have to accomplish.

17 Kick-start your thought process by listing all the possible solutions that come into your head, without judging whether they are good or bad.

18 Implement your solution by using the first item on your list. Continue the process until you find the solution that best fits the task.

19 Think about how good it feels when ideas flow.

20 Journal the experience of gaining clarity by focussing your thoughts on just one task.

21 Think about something you are close to achieving, specifically in the next few days. Imagine you have unlimited resources to complete this task.

22 Make a list of every point that needs to be covered to complete this goal.

23 Before implementing your plan, state to yourself that you will complete all of the items on your list by the end of the day.

24 Give yourself a special reward for having finished the task.

25 Journal how setting your intention to finish some-thing within a given time frame helped to complete the task.

26 Think about something you have always wanted but not yet achieved. This should be a general goal rather than a specific one.

27 Befriend someone who has already achieved your desire. Spend time discussing how they went about it and get excited about the process.

28 Draw up a practical 12-step action plan to put yourself in the right circumstances to achieve your goal.

29 Appreciate that it is the journey of achieving this goal that really matters.

30 Monitor your belief that your goal is achievable. Write down how you feel when progressing through each step of your plan. Remember, goals change.

| imagine | stimulate | create | appreciate | observe |

well done

Take the day to appreciate all that you have achieved in the last 30 days. See how it feels to let go of a few old ways of thinking.

Do something extra special today that makes you really happy and see how that feels. Give thanks to everyone that has helped you along the way to achieve your goals.

time to **reassess**

The lessons you need to learn in order to achieve your dreams are simple. See how many of the following methods you have started to use since reading this chapter.

Follow your heart

Let your inner wisdom guide you towards what you really want. When you open your heart, you are open to new ideas. You are able to let go of old ways of thinking in favour of new ideas that make you feel good on an inner level. Being true to yourself will get you wherever you want to go, and you will feel good in the process.

Dare to dream

Look at every possible solution to your problems by exercising all your senses and employing all the available creative methods. You will be amazed at what you can come up with when you simply let your ideas flow without judging them. Stimulating your imagination shows you all of your inner resources. Prioritise all your possible solutions according to what seems the easiest, quickest and most appropriate option.

Know what you want

Take an active role in deciding how your life will be by looking at what you want to gain from each situation: be conscious of your desires. Setting the stage for what you want, helps you to look for just those things. If you are looking for romance, you will find something in the situation

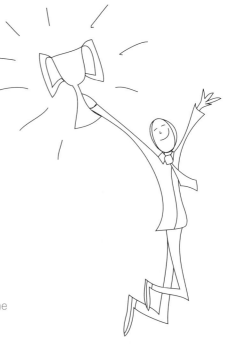

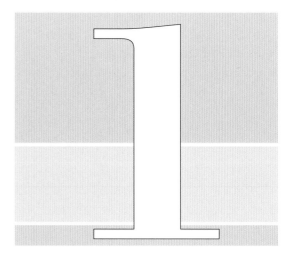

that's romantic to you. If you want laughter in everything you do, you will always find something funny. Know what you want, even for five minutes.

Use your powers of observation

Keep on top of all the signals – physical and emotional – that you receive daily to help keep you on the right path. Do a quick check of how you are feeling on the physical level. Are you looking after yourself? Are there things you do that make you feel great inside? Have you been learning new things or meeting new people? Write down as many interesting things that have happened over the last thirty days.

Be positive in all that you do

You get what you think about, whether you like it or not. Always focus your energy on looking forward towards the solution rather than back at the problem. When you do something positive for someone, it is reflected back at you.

Appreciate your achievements

Show gratitude for all that you have accomplished and everything around you. Programme your mind to believe only the best in you by repeating positive affirmations daily. Come to expect that you are the most deserving person in the world to achieve your dreams!

Understand where you are now

Working on your positive attitude changes you on all levels. The most obvious is how you feel physically, as physical stimulation immediately grabs your attention. When you feel hotter than normal, or are experiencing any discomfort, you know that you need to take action to remedy the situation. It makes you physically uncomfortable.

When you have an imbalance in your energy levels, you do not feel at your physical optimum. Being low in energy, can make you sluggish, lacking in enthusiasm and, eventually, physically unwell. Choosing to feel better empowers you to find the right combination of food, exercise and mental balance to achieve a perfect flow of energy throughout your mind, body and soul.

How have the effects of focussing your energy through the power of your positive thoughts changed your levels throughout the day? Go back and retake the Assess Your Energy Levels section of the Postive Behaviour Survey on pages 26–7. Check to see how your score has improved. Are there areas that you still need to work on? Use the exercises detailed in this chapter specific to your own progressive path.

If your energy levels are good, in all likelihood, you have seen the benefit derived from looking at things from a different perspective. Choosing to focus on what you want, rather than what you need, helps you become more aware of what you truly desire from every situation.

See how your attitude about yourself and others has changed by retaking the Assess Your Positive Power section of the Positive Behaviour Survey on pages 24–5. Are you happier as a result? Are you getting more done?

Now review the goals you set for yourself whilst working through the Achieve Your Dreams 30-day Action Plan. Did the exercise stimulate you mentally? Did you feel any differently towards the situation when you finished? If so, how did it feel? Were you able to concentrate? Did you achieve what you wanted and expected?

There is nothing better on this planet than understanding the true power that lies within you to explore your own unique place in the universe. It is only through the power of your thoughts that you get what you are thinking. Always make your thoughts a shining beacon, a great big banner to the universe that says 'this is what I really love to do or that I really want to be'.

have fun

I have a delightful story about one of my stepdaughters on her first day at school. When she got back home, we asked whether she had fun. She replied that it was funnier than she thought it would be. It is no coincidence that children have an innate ability to seek out the fun in many more situations than we do as adults. Sounds and smells, as well as things to touch and see, all provide great sources of joy and wonder when we are young. As a child, you are encouraged to use your imagination to explore the world. Your laughter is an indication that you are happy in your play with others, and with yourself.

As you grow older, you learn different rules of behaviour based on the specific activities you undertake. You are taught to be quiet in the library or classroom, for example, so that your attention can be focused on what you want to learn. Your family has its own set of rules governing the behaviour expected in the home. In some situations, you learn it is not acceptable to have fun at the same time as you are doing something else. This is the primary reason why many people hold the belief that it is not the done thing to have fun at work, during meals or whilst engaged in various other activities.

The truth is, you have to work at having fun! According to the principles of Dr. Usui – re-discoverer of the ancient healing system of Reiki – one of life's goals is to teach attitudes of enjoyment, health, happiness and light to the mind. By practising the skills of positive thinking, through your imagination and all of your senses, you become more aware of your inner feelings. Feeling enjoyment lets you know that you are connected to the moment and sensing the flow of energy throughout your body. When you are enjoying something, you feel alive physically, mentally and emotionally.

You can improve any situation by consciously choosing to get pleasure from the experience. The best way to achieve this is to pay attention to the things that you enjoy most. What can you do in each of your daily activities to bring more pleasure to the experience? Can you have more enjoyment from your morning shower, daily walk to work or regular evening meal? Can you gain satisfaction from your achievements during the day? Do you take the time to reward yourself for your efforts?

Given the option, you would choose to enjoy every part of your day, at work, with your partners or friends, and with family. You would choose to relax your body when you feel the desire, and take pleasure in each little experience of your day. There is absolutely nothing standing in your way. Learn to play.

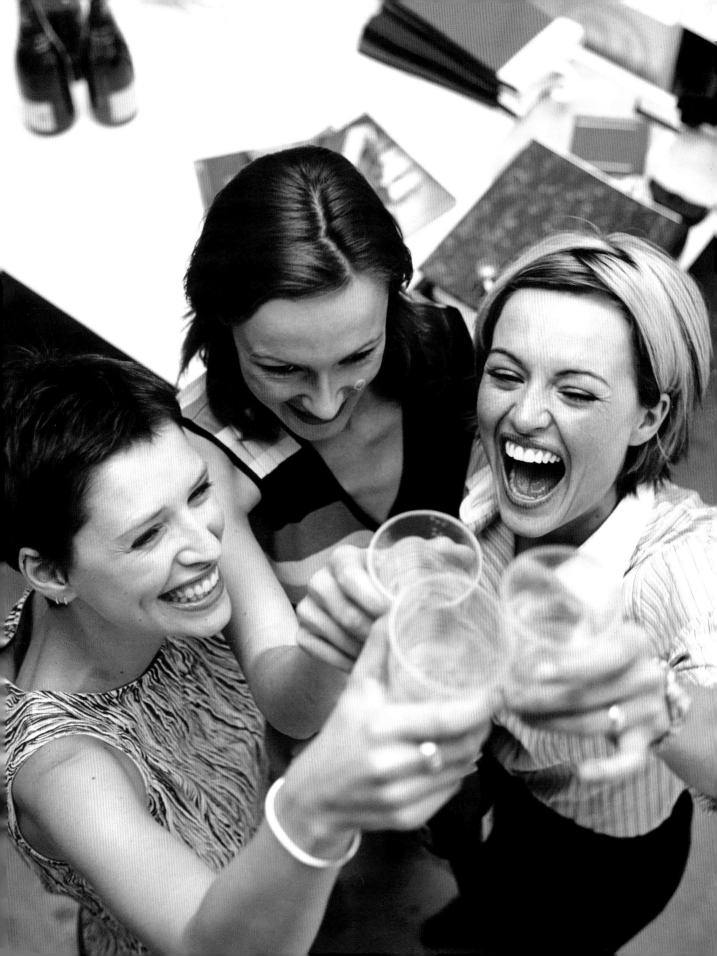

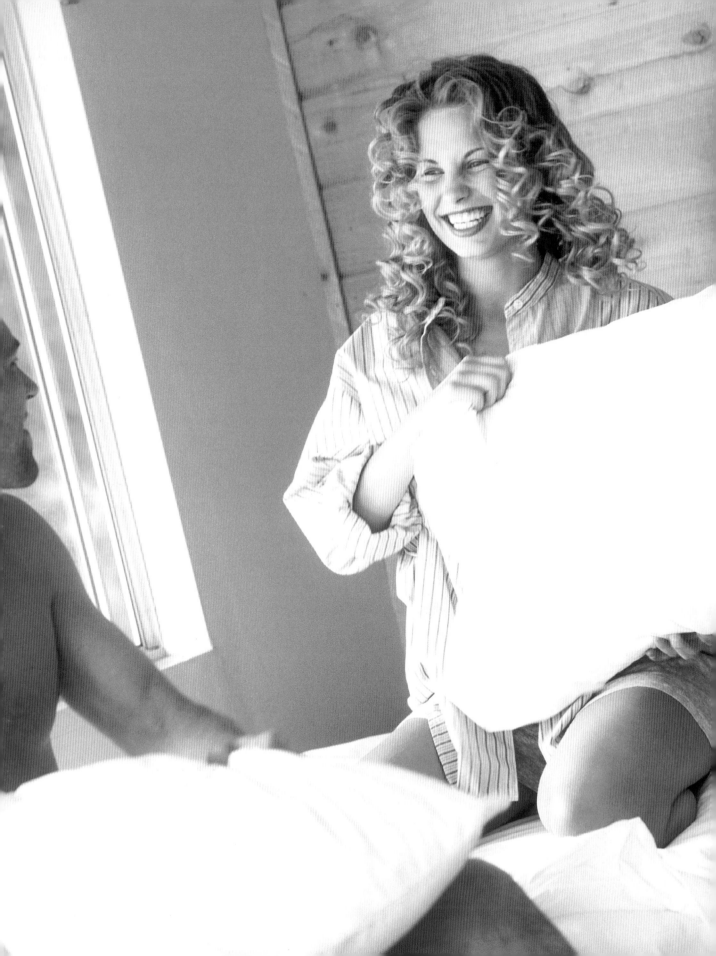

cherish intimate relationships

Intimate relationships are the most special, as you allow others to see your inner qualities, and in turn, you are allowed to see the inner qualities in others. You may have intimate relationships with many people, not just your partner. There may be members of your family, special friends or work colleagues who you relate to on a deeper level. In your intimate relationships, you hold a special place in your heart for the unique connection that you share with others.

To be intimate with another, you first need to be intimate with your own wants and desires. Knowing what lifts your soul to a higher place and expressing your inner excitement, enables you to attract others with similar passions. You are more likely to connect with someone on the same level if they are participating in something you too enjoy. Whatever you find interesting about your most treasured relationship needs to be nurtured throughout in order to keep the passion alive.

Sometimes you just cannot describe why you feel so attracted to someone, particularly when you have only recently met. Either it can seem as though you share many common likes and dislikes or you do not see eye-to-eye on anything at all, but feel a strong attraction on the physical level. Such attraction may be strong enough to last a lifetime or it may be only momentary in nature. Whatever the drawing power of the attraction, this type of relationship allows you to let go of your conscious thoughts that govern how you think you ought to behave, according to your pre-conceived notions,

and allow you to feel what is right in the moment. It taps into an inner level of consciousness that wants the freedom to express itself. For as long as each individual continues to feel recognition and appreciation for their spirit, the relationship will remain fun and uplifting.

In the early stages of involvement, perhaps before any real meaningful communication through words, you find ways of revealing more about your inner feelings. This is often done through the thoughtful selection of cards or gifts and or by writing messages that you find difficult to say out loud. As you become more confident that your feelings are shared, you engage in more revealing conversations and participate in joint activities that allow you to continue to expand and grow together. You indulge your imagination and think about ways of pleasing your partner and share your mutual passions.

Too often the day-to-day pressures of life put burdens on intimate relationships. Reality sometimes dampens the spirit. Putting the fun back into intimacy takes some time and effort, regardless of circumstances, to allow two souls re-unite. Ignite the flames of passion by dedicating time each day to have a laugh, to hold a conversation describing a great event in your day and to share one reason why you care for each other. It puts things in perspective and keeps the connection strong.

Antoine de Saint-Exupéry wrote, 'It is only with the heart that one can see rightly; what is essential is invisible to the eye.' I agree.

appreciate your loved ones

You can choose your friends, but you cannot choose your family, as the saying goes. Many Eastern cultures, however, believe that we do indeed choose our parents based on the lessons we need to learn in this lifetime.

Whatever your belief, the reality is most of us are brought up in a family structure that teaches us our earliest lessons in life. Much of your personality is formed by your interaction with your parents and siblings during early childhood, leaving you with a mixture of positive and negative attributes that you carry into your adult life.

As you get older, you scrutinise the knowledge you learnt as a child in the light of your own independent thoughts and feelings about your life experiences, and both accept and reject some of the values or principles that you learnt in childhood.

In all relationships, it is difficult not to take rejection on a personal level, so conflict can and does arise out of hurt feelings. Both learning to let go and learning to forgive are lessons that we all need to learn from our relationships with our family members.

Learn to be accepting

You cannot divorce yourself from your past, as you carry physical reminders of your parents through your genetic make-up. Your physical appearance, mannerisms and health are all a direct result of your birth circumstances. You carry your family name and all the associations of being part of your clan. You can carry the glory and sometimes the shame of your heritage.

It is the human condition that we all do things or have things done to us that we must learn to forgive and forget. Letting go of the hurt, anger and jealousies that may have formed during your upbringing is integral to moving forward in your life. You must learn to become accountable for your own behaviour and not blame the circumstances of your upbringing for areas of your life where problems exist. If old resentments are getting in the way of enjoying the positive feelings of being connected to someone, try the Open Your Heart Positive Action Exercise on pages 106–7.

Strengthen the bonds

Look for the best and ignore the rest is the right attitude to put the fun back into your family life. In all dealings with your family, choose to see only the things that you want to see, and you will feel the unconditional love permeate your inner being.

Like any intimate relationship, it will benefit from thoughtful gestures that recognise deeper connections. Making it a point to call with regularity, writing letters and celebrating occasions will go a long way towards making your family part of your life. Too often day-to-day pressures take precedence over keeping in touch with those we hold near and dear to our hearts. A five-minute phone call, a memorable card or a thoughtful letter takes only a few minutes but means more than you can imagine.

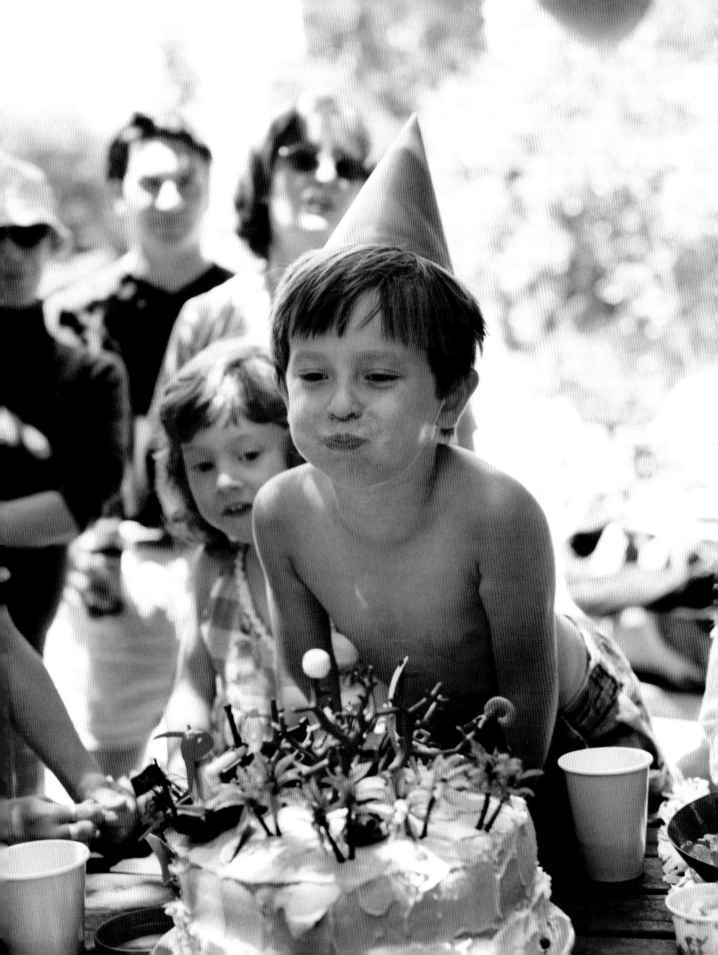

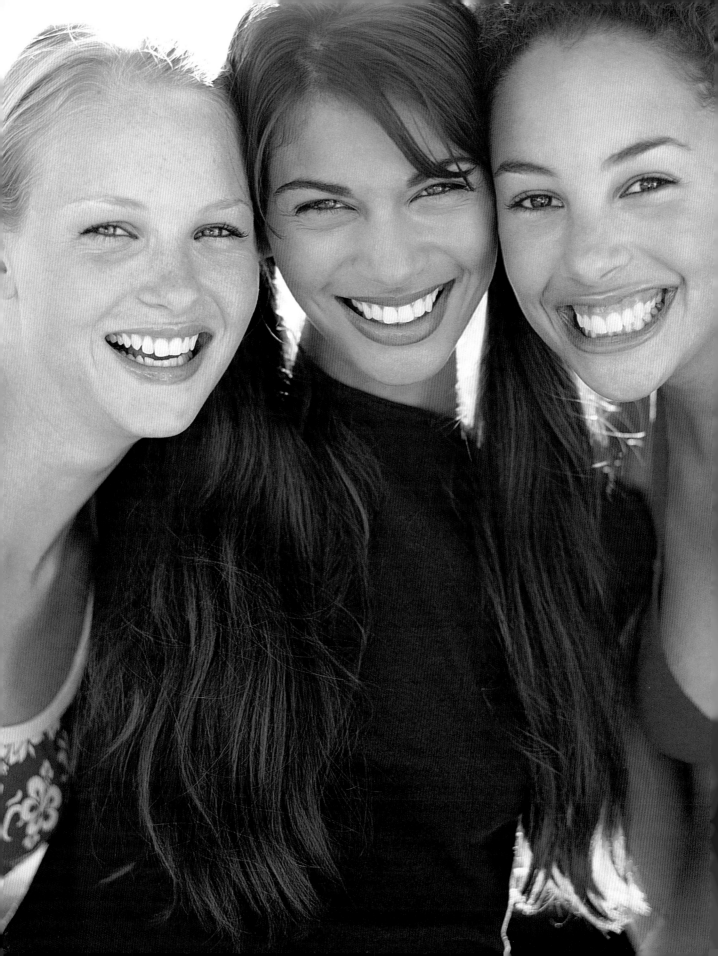

foster your friendships

Where would you be without your friends? They are there for you in times of need, joy and sorrow, and mostly, just the sound of their voice can bring sunshine to an otherwise dark and dreary day. Friends have the ability to make you laugh and bring out your human side. Special friendships, such as your intimate, physical or familal relationships, touch you at the very deepest levels of your soul. You allow your inner personality to be exposed, safe in the knowledge that your true friends will accept you as you are.

Friends add dimension to your life. You experience many things with your friends that you would be unlikely to experience on your own. You can pick up the phone and, in an instant, have companionship without even needing to say why. Your friends, most likely, cross many cultures and come from many areas, bringing a depth of knowledge that you would never gain without them. You have friends of many ages that help you to relate to life experiences. Most of all, your friends do not have to be identical in their thinking to you, making for stimulating and lively debate.

Be a good friend
Friendships transcend time and space and remain a part of your soul. We all think back fondly on the many friendships that we have enjoyed over the years, which seem only like yesterday. Whether a day or a decade passes without seeing each other, friends still have all the intimate moments shared together that never fade away.

Stay in touch
All too often, the pressures of everyday life take precedence over keeping in touch with those you hold near and dear to your heart. It only takes a few minutes to make a quick telephone call, scribble a memorable card or write a thoughtful letter, but these things can mean more than you might imagine. Think about your the friendships in your life that you may have let slip away. Say out loud that you are thinking of them. Do not be surprised if they are thinking about you at the same time.

Set aside one day a week to do something with a friend, without your partner. Interacting socially away from your day-to-day relationships, adds new experiences that you can eventually share with your partner. Treat your friends as you would like to be treated as a friend.

- Always honour secrets that you share, as friendship is a sacred trust

- Listen without judgement

- Give advise, only when asked

- Do not take your friends for granted

- Remember birthdays and special occasions

- Tell them how much you love them

As Ralph Waldo Emerson once wrote,
"The only way to have a friend, is to be one."

open your heart

>> positive action exercise

All too often, after our initial enthusiasm of becoming involved in a romantic relationship, we lose sight of our original attraction to our partners. All the time and energy that we spent thinking about the other person prior to a committed relationship, gets diverted when we begin to focus on the day-to-day business of dealing with the more mundane aspects of life. All too quickly our relationship can likewise become mundane.

Putting the fun back into your romantic relationship requires focussing your energy on what you want rather than need from your partnership. When you focus on what you need, you are concentrating your energy on what you do not have. What you find is that you get more of the same. When you turn your attention to what you desire, your enthusiasm and passion propels you forward to attracting that desire.

Taking positive action by looking at all the beneficial aspects of your relationship will help you to rekindle your initial attraction and move your relationship forward. We can all remember the moment when we realised that our love interest was mutual. The first time that we hear the words 'I love you' is a moment that stays with us forever. It is the essence of being accepted for who we are. We are happy and in a joyous state which makes all that we do seem to go more smoothly.

As our relationships progress, however, we often say 'I love you' as a matter of routine – words without emotion. To put the emotion back, we must look for the areas in which we can feel joy.

The feeling of joy triggers the body into producing endorphins – opium-like proteins naturally produced in our body. These hormones are responsible for creating physical feelings of well-being and, as a result, mental and emotional well-being. By learning to consciously trigger our body into producing endorphins, we can bring more enthusiasm and fun into our personal relationships.

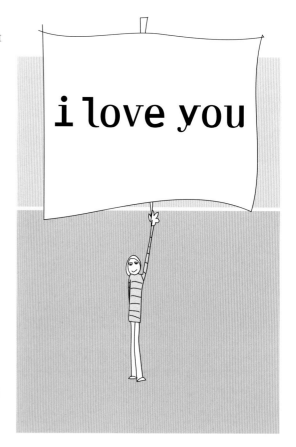

How do I love thee, let me count the ways

The following exercises are ways to concentrate on the positive aspects of your relationship with your partner. Practise them with an open mind and an open heart.

Think about the good times: one of the easiest and quickest ways to stimulate positive endorphins is to recreate an experience in your mind that was joyous. Think about your relationship with your partner and list the most joyous events that you have shared over the years, starting with the most recent. Try to list as many as possible.

Pick out the top five events on your list, the ones that make you the happiest, and describe them in detail. Try to be as descriptive as possible, remembering as much of the experience as you can, including where it occurred, what you were wearing, what the weather was like and whom you were with. Think about details such as music, colour, tastes, sights or smells that were part of the experience.

Now look closely at these five events to see if there are any similarities in the things that made you happy. You may find that whenever you are in a certain location you have shared a joyous moment. They could be triggered by eating a certain food, being with certain friends or occurring at a certain time of the day or year. Circle on your list all the elements these events had in common.

Ask your partner to make the same list of the most joyous events you have shared. Look at the elements that are the same but also note the differences in how each of you experience joy. Utilising the common experiences from your lists, start with those things that you and your partner find mutually joyful and plan to incorporate them into your current circumstances.

Communicate your thoughts

When we first fall in love, we tell everyone who is willing to listen about all of the wonderful attributes of the object of our affections. As our lives progress and we get busier and busier, we often fail to make the time to continue this process of communicating the things we most love about our companions. When we send positive signals to those we love, we make it safe for them to love us back. By elevating our relationship from the trivia of the mundane to the higher level of our spiritual connection or attraction, we are able to regain the intimacy that often gets lost over time.

Focus your attention on the things you love most about your partner. To do this sit down and write them a love letter concentrating on all of their positive attributes. Be as descriptive as you can. Think about how they affect all of your senses – sight, smell, touch, sound, taste and your sixth sense of intuition, your inner knowing.

Change your habits

We are all guilty of falling into the same routines with our partners. The pressures of work and family life often mean that the amount of time we devote to our intimate relationships lessens as our partnerships progress.

Put the zing back into your relationship by making a list of all of the activities you did at the beginning of your relationship that no longer play a part in your life together now. These may include going to the cinema, participating in sports, cooking for friends or disappearing together on the spur of the moment. Write down when you last did each activity.

Pick a few of these activities that you both enjoyed most and do them over the next six weeks. By changing our routines to be more stimulating and exciting, we can keep the relationship moving forward in a positive direction.

plan a memorable event

>> positive action exercise

Show your appreciation for your most intimate relationships by planning a special day to let them know how much you care.

Make the effort

Whether organising an intimate dinner for two or a party for many, the more time and effort you put into the planning, the more likely you will be able to implement details that will touch those that you care about. Begin by thinking about the following:

Timing. The more people on your guest list, the longer lead time you will need. For big events that involve gathering people from out of town, try to send invitations out at least two months in advance. Smaller parties with a more local guest list should be given one month's notice. If you are planning a more intimate dinner for two, try making it a surprise!

Venue. Get sentimental and think of a place with meaning to those you want to feel special. Think about the location of special events that have taken place in their life and show them that you remember the significance. Plan for all eventualities such as weather, ease of transportation and always send detailed directions with the invitation.

Menu. Think about the significant meals that you have shared together and incorporate favourite foods into the menu. If you are preparing the food yourself, make sure to plan extra time to have everything finished before your guests arrive.

The most important part of the party is to spend time with those you love.

Titillate the senses

First impressions always count, so make sure the invitations are very special and, when you are guests arrive, they are knocked out by all they see.

Get creative. Think about using a special photograph that you can mount on a piece of lovely paper with a personal handwritten note inside, or perhaps a greeting card that has special relevance. Look at every detail down to the stamps that you select. Little details go a long way.

Set the tone. Fragrance and lighting are essential to creating atmosphere for your special event. Special flowers or scents that have meaning will show how attentive you are to their innermost feelings. Candles always creative an intimate atmosphere, so make sure you have plenty on hand.

Seranade your guests. Music elevates the soul, so pay special attention to the music that you select. Think about music that will have special poignancy and be sure to select the music for the evening in advance of the event.

Commemorate the day. Be sure to take lots of photographs. Leave disposable cameras around for everyone to capture the event. Send the best ones to your loved ones to make the day memorable.

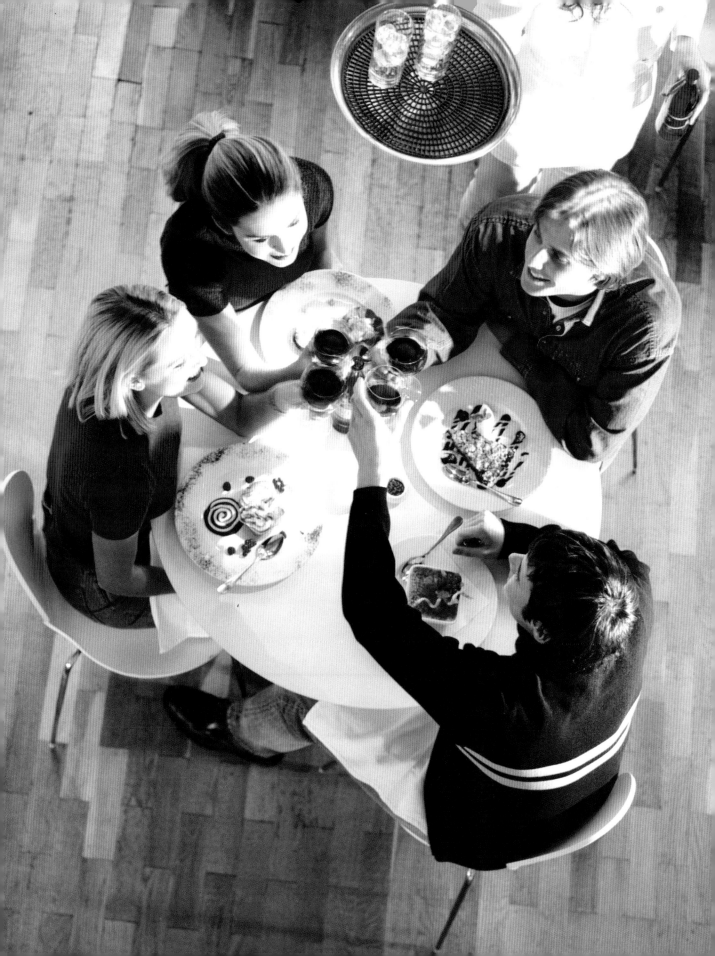

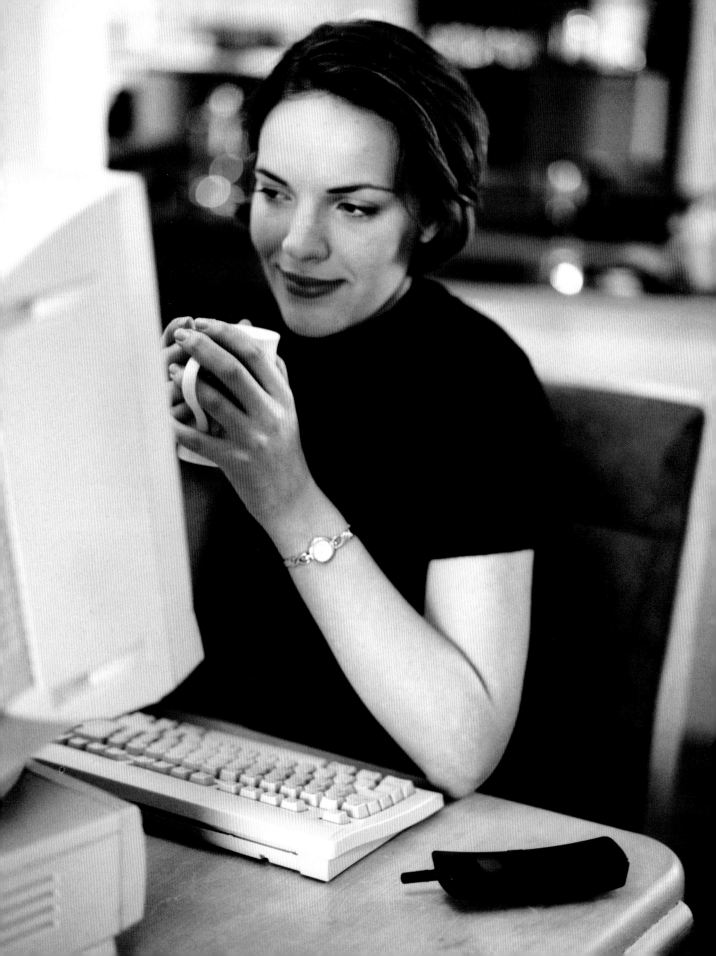

whistle while you work

We spend up to one third of our lives working, which is a substantial chunk of the time we have on this earth. It is entirely up to you how enjoyable an experience you make it. How much positive energy you put into your chosen career will, without exception, make the experience more pleasant. Simply by focussing your attention on doing the best you can in each situation, you will feel a greater sense accomplishment and contentment in the workplace.

Choose a career, not just a job

To begin with, it is essential to understand what you want to gain from your employment. Most people would probably answer that they need to work in order to support their lifestyle. While this is an honest response, placing the emphasis on *needing* a job rather than *wanting* a career, makes you feel more tense about the situation. As you will recall from earlier chapters, concentrating on the need focusses on the lack of something and brings about negative feelings. It is very difficult to relax and have fun when you feel that everything you do may threaten your livelihood.

Considering all the benefits you desire from your work experience will help you to prioritise the best approach to achieve your desired results. Aside from the financial reward, what are the reasons that you are working in your current career? Think about the following reasons, and add your own personal statements to this list:

- To gain independence
- To challenge your mind
- To become successful
- To meet new people
- To learn new skills
- To develop your creative skills
- To prove you can do it
- To express your passion

The best way to have fun and truly whistle while you work is to fulfil your intentions from your work experience and focus your attention on these goals. All too often, you get caught up in all of the personality conflicts that may arise when working with many people. Rather than taking action and doing the things you are responsible for to the best of your abilities, you spend your time looking at who got what from whom. You conveniently place the control in the hands of others, your bosses or co-workers, rather than taking responsibility for your own actions.

No matter how mindless the tasks are that you are required to do, give them your undivided attention. If you put your heart and soul into it, both your heart and soul will be nourished by the experience. One third of your life can be a lot more fun just by following this simple advice.

atmosphere makes a difference

You may be unable to control many elements of your work environment, including the location, size and shape of your workspace. How you feel physically when you are in your office, unit or other work environment makes a huge difference to how much you accomplish. Despite the type of space, however, there are things you can do to feel more comfortable.

Atmosphere is not just about the room you inhabit, the air you breathe or the cosmetic touches of your office, it is how the space makes you feel when you walk in through the door. Many factors affect an atmosphere, but mostly it is created by the inhabitants of the space. Tranquil environments usually house peaceful and calm people. Creative environments play home to lots of stimulating objects and highly energetic people, whilst stressed environments house tense and unhappy people.

You cannot change your co-workers without changing your job, so if you enjoy your work but find that some people make the atmosphere in the office uncomfortable, you must learn to see only the things that you desire whenever you walk through the door.

Establish a mini-climate

Adjust your workspace to make yourself more comfortable. Bring attitudes and objects that help you to feel jolly and relaxed into your personal work area, regardless of what is going on elsewhere. Imagine that in your space, you rule the roost. You are entirely responsible for every word that you say and all the work that is required of you. This space will be used only for positive thoughts and actions, and no one can influence your attitudes or moods whilst you are in your own area. Whenever you enter, imagine that your workspace is protected by a great golden light.

Take notice of how you feel. We are all entitled to have the essentials that make our work experience a comfortable one. If any of them are lacking, ask your boss to help remedy the situation. Pay attention to the following and see how they feel:

- If you sit at a desk, is your chair comfortable?
- Do you have adequate lighting?
- Is the temperature comfortable most times?
- Does it seem noisy?
- Do you have any safety concerns?

Once you have attended to the basics, look at other ways to feel good in your space. Even if your desk is in an open-plan office, which can leave little room for privacy, create an atmosphere that is conducive to the way that you work. You must be able to focus your attention on what is required of you, so create the best atmosphere to keep your mind on getting the task done. It is all too easy to get involved in everyone else's jobs when working in close confines.

Most people fall into one of two categories – creative right-brain thinkers or logical left-brain thinkers. Someone with a logical approach may find a creative office atmosphere off-putting, whereas someone with a creative mind may find it difficult to create in an atmosphere where things are too logical.

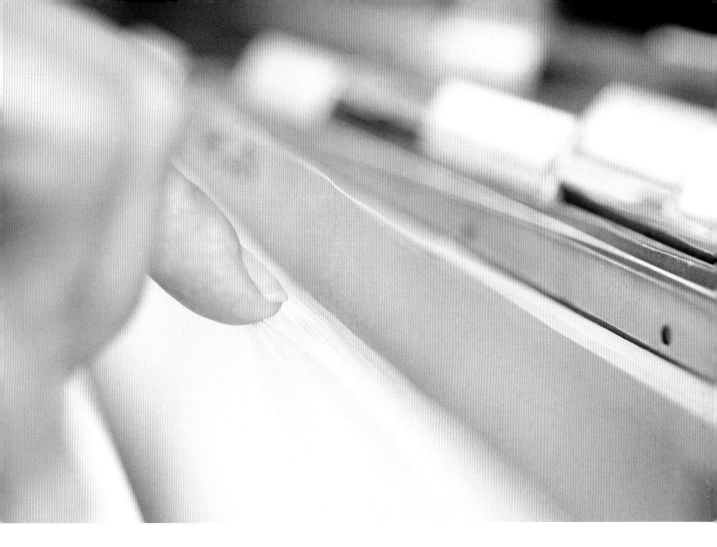

Creative spaces incorporate many things to stimulate the senses. The creative spaces that I have worked in were far less structured, chaotic and contained more objects than found in a more logical space. A larger work surface is usually required to accommodate the things that inspire creative minds.

In creative spaces, magazine cuttings and other reference materials can provide stimulation, along with work in progress, samples and materials, but all this can take up quite a bit of space. Go through all of the items you have collected. Review all your magazines and reduce them by 25 percent. Too much stimulation can divert your attention from your own creativity. To stay fresh and better focus your energy, have a good clear out of your space every few months. If you hold on to too many old ideas, there is not much room for new inspirations.

Logical spaces suit logical thinkers who require a less stimulating space with fewer distractions. If you are a logical worker in a space that doesn't work for you, it will be very difficult to accomplish your goals efficiently. To feel most comfortable in an open environment, you may want to use your computer or other large items to create more of an enclosed space to remove yourself from the office chatter.

To make the most of your atmosphere, the more systems you are able to put in place, the easier it will be to access the materials you need which will help you to feel in control of your space. Keeping all surfaces free from clutter at the end of each day will enable you to structure your day more efficiently and stay focused on what you need to achieve on a daily basis.

get the buzz

Isn't it terrific when you really get into doing what you set out to and things seem to fall into place? You get into the spirit and concentrate your energy on that one particular thing and work it through to completion. When you finish the task, you feel really good about yourself, physically excited and stimulated. You do not have to be creating a masterpiece. Any task that needs doing, even the washing up, can give you an inner buzz.

Undertaking every project with enthusiasm will, I guarantee, make each and every job more fun, even the most repetitive and mundane task. Enthusiastic people are always up for it, and ready to give anything their best go. They have a positive attitude and embody the philosophy that nothing ventured, is nothing gained. You will probably notice that enthusiastic people are fun to be around. They motivate you to look on the bright side and often times, they bring you along for the ride. Everything is much more fun when you give it your best go.

Be your own cheerleader

In America, every sporting event is accompanied by cheerleaders – a group of enthusiastic supporters who motivate their team through chanting out loud. The crowd enthusiasm for any event impacts on the performance of those participating. We have all appreciated the benefits of encores from entertainers who enjoyed the interaction with their audience. Try out this exercise on at least one project each day for the next week, and see what a difference it makes.

Imagine that you are a cheerleader, encouraging and supporting yourself in your own efforts. You are always at your side chanting words of encouragement. Although you may feel silly to begin with, keep doing it throughout the project. Try these out and see how they make you feel:

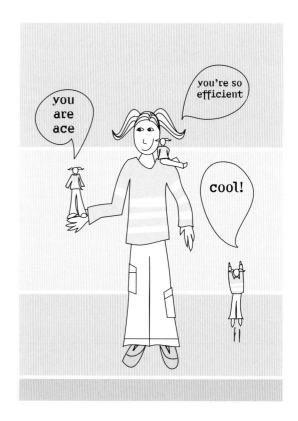

- You are the best

- You are brilliant at your job

- You are the most accurate at what you do

- You are very creative

- You are a great communicator

- You get things done efficiently

- You are very speedy at what you do

Give your undivided attention to the task in hand. If you are enthusiastic, you will find nothing else going on around you really matters. You do not get restless or find yourself distracted by noise; you get into the rhythm of it and let yourself go for it. Doing your best, is the best thing you can do.

Find your true passion

Some people know their chosen vocations from an early age. Such strength of vision is usually an indication that you are aware of your innate talents. If spotted at a young age, talent can be nurtured and encouraged to reach its maximum potential.

Most of us, however, try our hand at many things before we get excited, and settle on something that utilises our talents. Each new job you turn your hand to adds another set of skills to your cumulative knowledge and teaches you valuable lessons about your strengths and weaknesses. It is as important to learn about the things that you do not like as well as the things that bring you pleasure to truly create the ideal working situation.

Sometimes you are afraid to express where your true passion lies, in fear that you may not be good enough to pursue it as an option. You may also fear social pressure from those around you to not take risks and try to achieve your innermost dreams. In reality, by following your passion, you will always find ways to get what you really want.

Many of us are guilty of finding excuses to not do what we really want. By doing this you

sabotage your ability to make it happen. Having faith in your ability to unlock your hidden talents and spread them into the universe, is the only necessary requirement to make things happen. Deep, down inside we all know the things we are meant to be doing. They make you feel good just thinking about them.

List ten professional achievements you would like to gain and that you believe you have the talent to accomplish. List them in priority of importance, beginning with the one thing that you would really like to strive for. If you have already accomplished some of your goals, write the date next to the achievement.

_____ _____

_____ _____

_____ _____

_____ _____

_____ _____

_____ _____

_____ _____

_____ _____

_____ _____

_____ _____

Next, list all the skills and experience you have accumulated throughout your career that will enable you to get to where you want to be. Think of each job and all the different skills that you acquired

Compare where you are now with where you want to be. Make a list of the steps you need to take you from A to B. There may be one or one hundred, the number does not matter. Look for the small steps you can take to realise your inner desire. Being in the right place at the right time is just a matter of seeking out life's opportunities. Decide what feels right in your heart and do not worry about the consequences. You will always be led in the right direction.

take a break

We can all reap the benefit of taking some time out from an arduous work schedule. Taking a breather, by stepping away from a task that seems difficult to accomplish, can refresh and invigorate your mind and get your creative juices flowing again. Even a few minutes of absorbing new and exciting stimuli can help you to view your job from a new perspective.

Get out more

By the laws governing employment, those of us who do not work for ourselves but are employed by either a company or an individual are entitled to take at least three breaks a day – a short break in the morning and afternoon, and a lunchbreak that is usually an hour long. For many workers, a normal break consists of having a quick cup of something whilst chatting with a group of colleagues. Although this can be a great way of strengthening your ties with co-workers, this time is often used as an impromptu session to gripe about all of the negative aspects of what is going on in the workplace. See what a difference a change of routine can make in getting your work done efficiently.

Break the habit. For the next week, each time you have a few spare minutes away from your desk, leave your workplace, even if only for fifteen minutes. Make it a point to physically leave the office for each of your breaks during the day.

Try a different activity each day from following list. See how different you feel on your return.

| Sit outside a cafe and people watch

| Read a newspaper or magazine

| Go for a walk in the nearest green space

| Meditate for fifteen minutes

| Plan a lunch with friends rather than colleagues

| Go window-shopping

| Go to a museum or exhibition and get inspired

Let go of your rigid ways of thinking and open yourself up to new ideas. Each new experience you have in your life brings an added dimension to your work. Welcome new experiences each day by consciously deciding to have them. Make a positive affirmation that says: 'Each day I embrace all change that will enable me to have new ideas.'

Change your work schedule

As with most things in life, work becomes routine and, as a consequence, it is easy to lose enthusiasm. This makes it difficult to complete projects. One way to break the cycle is to turn your day upside down. Look at ways to change the times that you undertake activities, arrange meetings at different times of the day and schedule in thinking time to give your mind the chance to seek new ideas.

Set your intention to discover new ideas or ways to solve a problem. Like a positive affirmation, ask out loud for the specific knowledge that you wish to

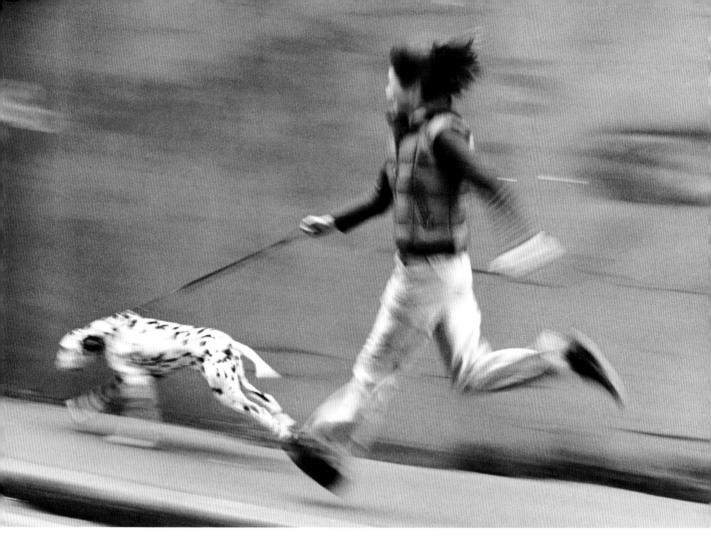

gain such as, 'I would really like to know the best way to do —'. Now forget about it, just have the expectation that the information will come to you.

Return to the issue that you were thinking about and list ten ways to deal with the problem. It does not matter how silly the ideas sound, just write them down. It is easy to get into a rut when trying to figure out ways to sort through an issue. You can think so hard about the problem that you forget to consider the solutions.

Continue listing all the conceivable solutions until you cannot think of another thing. Number each in order, with the easiest and quickest solution to the problem first. Now take action. Keep working through your list until you have solved the problem.

Develop your career

Most companies will support an employee's career growth. Take control of your own professional development by looking for ways of learning new skills, such as taking a training course, that will make your job more enjoyable. You will not get things if you do not ask for them, so think about what knowledge would help you make your job easier. Research where and when the course is available, then ask your company if they will pay for the course. You will probably find they are supportive.

Time away in a new, exciting environment can stimulate your mental capacity and inject enthusiasm into your professional life. Being willing to learn more shows those around you that you are interested in your job and are keen to progress along your career path. It is a win-win situation.

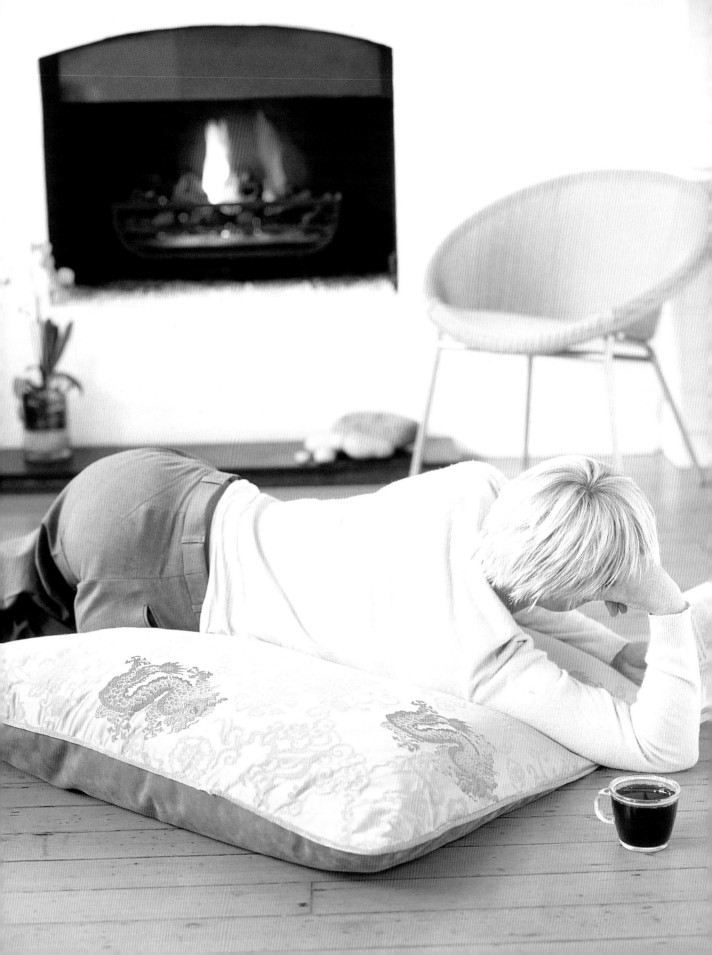

lie back and relax

Making the time each day for relaxation is integral to maintaining physical, mental and emotional health. Your physical body, mind and soul need a rest from the pressures and responsibilities of your daily routine. Learning to disengage from constant physical and mental activity allows you to release any tension, which can in some cases lead to physical, mental and emotional dis-ease.

When you are stressed, your body signals to you that it is time to slow down and chill out. Common ailments associated with stress, such as high blood pressure, headaches and chest pains, can lead to more serious medical problems, such as heart disease and a mental or emotional breakdown. It is no coincidence that these symptoms occur in the areas of the head and the heart, centres of both thoughts and emotions. If you are experiencing any stress-related illnesses, it means that what you are thinking about at that moment is not in your best interests. You only have one body for the duration of your life, so learning to slow down and relax is an important factor in leading a healthier and longer life.

Take a deep breath

You can easily learn ways of relaxing. One of the simplest and quickest methods is to practise controlled breathing. Breathing is an automatic physical function that we all do naturally, without thinking, and so take for granted. However, when you are tense, your breathing tends to be shallower, which prevents oxygen from fully reaching your brain. When experiencing stress, you raise your shoulders, putting strain on and tension into the neck. This can be painful and is often difficult to ignore. In extreme cases, such as a panic attack, you can hyperventilate – or breathe too quickly with short, shallow breaths. This is often followed by an elevated heartbeat that can feel like your heart is jumping out of your body. The quickest way to sort out these symptoms is to take more controlled breaths. Other common methods are meditation, yoga, physical exercise or reading, which all allow you to concentrate your attention in a positive way on your mind, body and spirit.

Do not disturb

You may have your own favourite way to relax. You can often trigger your body into a relaxed state just by envisaging the perfect escape. This is a personal reaction, as what is calm and relaxing for you, may be terrifying for someone else. Think about your favourite ways of finding relaxation and, even if you are unable to find the time to retreat, you can still create the visual picture in your mind's eye and gain the same benefits. A minimum of twenty minutes relaxation a day will help to keep you physically, mentally and emotionally fit.

A relaxed body and mind make it easier to connect to what is going on around you. When you are tense and living too much inside your head, you are often unable to see the signs that will point you in the right direction. It is a constantly downward spiral.

strive for harmony

We all share the ability to bring our bodies into a harmonious state of being by listening to the requirements of our mind, body and spirit. When you feel out of sorts, either physically or emotionally, it is often because you are failing to acknowledge some aspect of your being.

When a choir sings in harmony, there are many different voices, all singing different parts, that combine to make the song sound whole. An individual part sung alone, however, does not have the balance of the upper, lower and middle notes that makes it harmonious to the ear. As in music, when you, as an individual, fulfil your physical, mental, emotional and spiritual needs in every task that you undertake, your being feels integrated, healthy, balanced and whole.

Get a tune up

One of the greatest ways to get tuned up and become one with your body is to take up some form of physical exercise that you commit to practising several times a week. Try to develop a routine that you repeat on the same days each week. Try not to miss out a day, unless it is really unavoidable. Remember that it takes just six weeks to form a habit. Keep the routine going and it will soon become something that you look forward to doing each week.

All forms of physical exercise bring added awareness to your physical being. In the process, you are able to let go of your unwanted thoughts and day-to-day worries and become more intimately acquainted with how your body is responding to your current lifestyle. Regular practice makes you feel and look better and dramatically improves your feelings of self-worth. The release of endorphins into your system that come with regular exercise brings an added benefit in feelings of well-being.

Many practices such as yoga, t'ai chi, and qi gong are physical regimes that work not only on your physical body, but also on your mental and spiritual levels. They affect the energy centres, or chakras, that we all have running throughout our bodies. These same energies are harnessed through the power of the mind in many forms of spiritual healing. I would highly recommend this combination approach to help you to become more aware of your full potential. Once you master the ability to feel energy flowing throughout your body, you will be more aware when blockages arise. You can release the blocks using the Postive Action Exercises in each chapter of this book.

Hum out loud

Start your day by humming a tune. Humming is a great way to raise your physical vibration and get all parts of your body working on the same level. Do this for five minutes every morning. After your humming session, make a positive affirmation out loud, stating that your body is in a natural and harmonious state of being. In each thing that you do, try to get your body, mind and inner self all singing from the same hymn sheet.

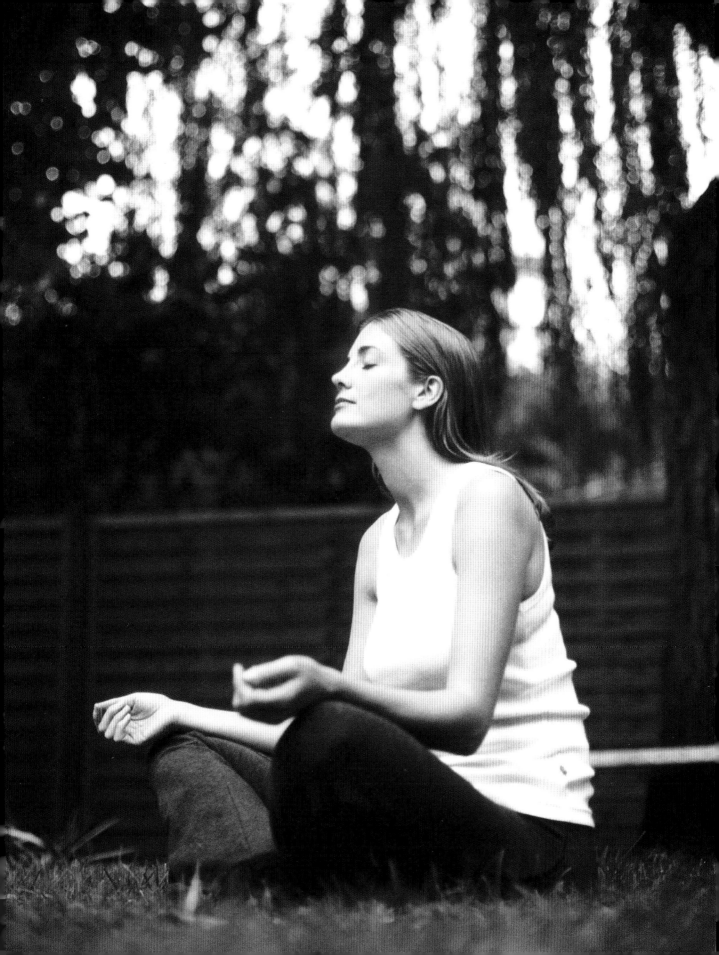

calm your mind

Many of the things done for relaxation do not completely relax the mind. You may choose to read a book or relax in front of the television, but all too often thoughts of the day still pop into your head. You may even physically feel the strain in your neck and shoulders from all the tensions of the day. The only true way to relax is to learn to accept that there may be unfinished matters to attend to, but it does not really matter in the moment. You can learn various methods of letting go of your thoughts for the present moment, and give your mind a break.

Clear your mind

Meditation is a method of calming the mind by releasing all thoughts. It is a great way to both start and end each day; life is so much more enjoyable when you are relaxed.

Very few of us breath properly, but you can create stress in your neck and shoulders by not consciously paying attention to your breathing. The physical benefits of breath-counting meditation lie in utilising your diaphragm muscle and increasing your lung capacity. Like all muscles, the diaphragm needs to be exercised properly.

Get up thirty minutes earlier than usual for the next week and start your day by clearing and expanding your mind. You can do this exercise whilst in bed, although it is sometimes easy to fall asleep and not gain the full benefit. I suggest sitting in a comfortable chair with your feet on the ground and your spine pressed up against the back of the chair.

Close your eyes and focus on your breathing. The objective here is to clear your mind of all other thoughts and concentrate only on your breathing. Allow any thoughts that enter your mind to pass right by, as if resting on a big fluffy cloud that floats away to return at another time. To help concentrate your thoughts, use the word 'one' when you breathe in and 'two' when you breathe out.

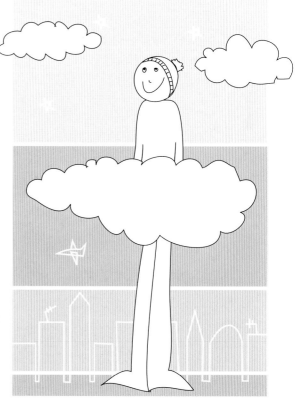

Let your thoughts go. When you begin this practice, you may find many thoughts keep coming into your head. Do not worry about it, simply go back to saying the word 'one' when you take a breath in, then 'two' when you take a breath out. Resist the temptation to move about, simply return your thoughts to the breathing process. After a while, you will forget about everything and find yourself in a very peaceful place. Stay there for twenty minutes.

Slowly bring your attention back to your physical body. Before you open your eyes, wriggle your toes and feel your feet firmly on the ground. In your own time, gradually open your eyes and gently move your body, paying attention to your arms, shoulders and head.

Create a mental retreat

Another method of calming the mind is through creative visualisation. Wouldn't it be lovely if you were able to escape to your favourite place each time you needed some relaxation? By using your imagination, you can create a personal relaxation retreat, that combines elements of all your favourite spaces. You can retreat here daily to give your body and most importantly, your mind, some time out.

Your mental retreat will be a place you can use to refresh and cleanse your mind on a daily basis. The more time you spend thinking about the personal details that you would like in your space, the more interesting you will find the experience. Do this exercise at home in your personal space, or take time out from work and find your favourite outdoor space to enjoy a mental break.

Start with the breath-counting meditation to relax your body. Wear loose clothing and sit in a comfortable chair.

Think of a place you find magical and relaxing. It could be somewhere by the sea, in the woods, up a mountain or a spa that you have visited in the past. Wherever you choose, try to capture all the elements that make you feel good.

Wash away your cares. Before you enter your retreat, begin by washing away everything that has happened during the course of the day. Think about how wonderful it feels to be freshly washed and dressed. Imagine relaxing in a magnificent bathtub with aromatic oils, having a wonderful shower, or swimming in the sea. Create some luxurious towels ready to warm you after your cleansing process, then put on the most comfortable clothing you can imagine.

Enter your personal retreat. Imagine that you're the only person ever allowed in your special place. Because you have created a perfect vision of this space, everything that you desire is already there. Walk into your space and take a look around at all the relaxing ways you can spend your time. What's the temperature like? Are you all wrapped up in toasty clothing or basking in the hot sunshine with barely anything on? What kinds of scents can you smell? What colours stand out in your mind?

Spend twenty minutes exploring and truly enjoying your space. Take off your shoes. Think about how it feels to walk on the ground or floor. Is it hot or cold? What sounds can you hear? If you want to sit down, think about where you would like to perch. How does it feel? You can change any detail at any time, so if you find that something does not tickle your fancy, simply imagine something else.

Slowly bring your attention back to where you are in the present moment, once you have truly enjoyed spending time in your space and feel your body relaxed all over. Wiggle your toes and gently move your body whilst you gradually open your eyes. You will feel better for your break and in the knowledge that you can return to your retreat anytime you choose.

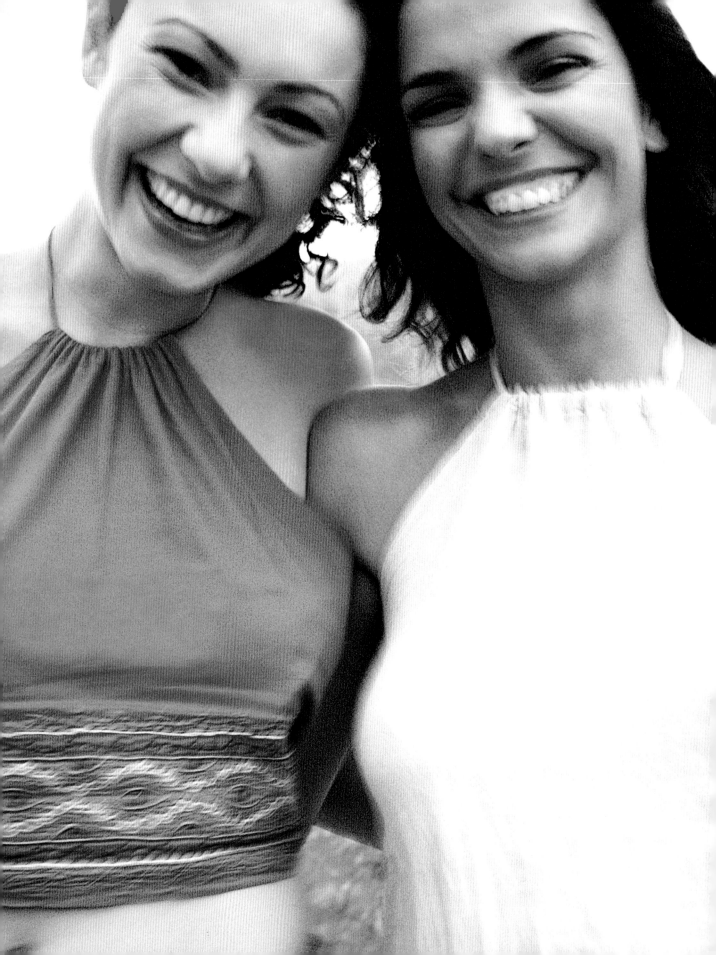

ha ha ha game

>> positive action exercise

When I was a child, my friends and I used to amuse ourselves by playing the Ha Ha Ha Game. One person would start by saying 'Ha'. The next person would then have to add another 'Ha' and so on, until someone fell out laughing! We rarely were able to get past 'Ha, ha, ha' without the entire group bursting into fits of giggles. Laughter and smiles are contagious and are universally understood throughout the world.

Laughter is a great way of releasing excess tension and negative energy from your body. When you laugh or smile, you raise your spirit and look at things with a much more positive outlook and you become far more approachable to others. You are much more likely to get what you want out on any situation when you start with a smile on your face.

Put on a happy face

To see how a smile can instantly change the way you look and feel, take a look at yourself in a mirror without smiling. Now put a smile on your face and see what happens. What changes do you see in your physical appearance? Do your eyes take on a sparkle? Does it make you feel better inside?

Make the conscious decision to smile each time you come in contact with another person, regardless of the situation, for the next week, to see how your smile impacts on those around you. At the end of the day, note the following observations in your journal:

Did you make more eye contact with those around you?

Were you more aware of things going on around you?

Did you engage in more conversations?

Were you able to get what you wanted in each situation?

Did you feel more relaxed?

Did people smile back?

You will mostly likely discover that people are more receptive to you when you have a smile on your face.

Quick-fix laughter toolkit

Put together a laughter toolkit for whenever you need a quick boost of giggles. Any time you feel yourself getting a bit tense, pick your favourite remedy to get you out of the doldrums. Add anything to the list that always makes you laugh.

Buy five funny videos

Write down your five favourite jokes and keep them with you

Get someone to tickle you

Take a trip to the zoo

Remember five of the funniest things that have ever happened to you

30-day action plan

The best way to enjoy life is by finding fun in all you do. When you look for humour, amusement and adventure in each experience, you allow yourself the freedom to laugh at your failures and explore the world by looking for things that make you feel good. Use the 30-day action plan to inject some spirit into your relationships, gain inspiration and enjoyment from your career path and plan activities to let your hair down and truly relax your body and soul.

goal	imagine	stimulate	create	appreciate	observe
spend more time sharing interests in an intimate relationship	**1** When you first met, what inner connection made your souls sing? Think about your common interests when you last did them together.	**2** Remember your friend in as much detail as possible. Write down five things that make them laugh, they love to do and make them sad.	**3** Plan a special day out. Walk in an inspirational place. Have a meaningful conversation. Plan their favourite meal. Do things together you both enjoy.	**4** Whether you live together or apart, find the perfect card or write a handwritten letter expressing all that they bring to your life.	**5** How does your heart feel when you make someone happy? Write down any changes in your relationship caused by showing an interest in your friend.
improve upon a family relationshp	**6** Pretend you were best friends growing up. Think about all the things you have in common and imagine doing something that you both enjoy.	**7** Go through old photos of your relative. Look for snaps that reflect a happy moment. Make a list of all this person has done for you from their heart.	**8** Let go of old grievances. Find neutral ground, pick up the phone and invite them back into your life. Commemorate your meeting with a photo.	**9** Be thoughtful. Follow up your meeting with a letter to show your appreciation for the time you spent together.	**10** How has the relationship changed by treating your relatives as your best friend. Are they more supportive in your life? Caring is a two-way street.
enlist colleagues to try a new approach at work	**11** You lack the confidence to try something new. Imagine colleagues have three positive things to say about your idea. Listen to their good points.	**12** To co-create, every group member needs to participate. Consider individual strengths. Ask for input from everyone to add excitement to the project.	**13** Write a mission statement on how the idea will benefit your work environment. Credit individuals for their ideas. Share it among your colleagues.	**14** Interact with others to gain inspiration. Work for a common outcome to unite minds. Consider five ways someone in your professional life adds to your day.	**15** Develop confidence by trying out ideas. For a week, let people in and see what they think. Write down ideas without judging them. See what you learn.

20
What do you want to achieve whilst having fun? Write down all ideas without judgement. Are they funnier than you thought?

25
Before a tense situation, take 17 seconds to relax. Choose to see things that make you comfortable. Write down your positive thoughts on the situation.

30
Clear your mind of clutter. Do your sleep patterns change? Write down your dreams. Gain insight on issues that are easier resolved when relaxed.

observe

appreciate

19
Life is full of contrasts. Adding fun to a chore makes it go more quickly. Feel the stress melt away when you find ways to have a laugh.

24
Relax your body each day, if only for 15 minutes. Feel the energy flowing without any blockages. Remember what it feels like.

29
Experience the calm that relaxation brings. Let unwanted thoughts drift away on fluffy white clouds. Feel the peace and serenity within.

create

18
See how many ways you can do the job and have a laugh: sing a funny song or wear silly clothes. Set a time limit and treat yourself when you finish.

23
Imagine a golden light bathing your body in unconditional love. As it washes over your body, imagine tension flowing out through your feet.

28
Practice a relaxation technique nightly. Also, once a week, set aside two hours of uninterrupted time to give yourself a special pampering.

stimulate

17
Think about all the silly ways you have tried to accomplish this chore in the past, and have a good laugh at yourself. Find humour in the situation.

22
Control your breathing. Sit in a comfortable chair. Hold a deep breath to the count of seven, then exhale to the count of seven. Repeat three times.

27
List all scents, foods, colours, sounds and places you find relaxing. Put together a mental relaxation toolkit that can cue your body to relax.

imagine

16
Consider something you are required to do but find dull. Pretend you are a games maker and write a set of rules. Make laughter an integral part.

turn a work chore into a fun game

21
Consider your favourite spot where you can relax. Picture it in as much detail as possible. Imagine all the things you find relaxing there.

learn to relax your body in a tense situation

26
Imagine taking a relaxing bath with aromatherapy oils. Relax and rest your mind. When you empty the tub, imagine all your worries washing away

develop a relaxation regime

goal

well done
Take the day to appreciate all that you have achieved in the last 30 days. See how it feels to let go of a few old ways of thinking. See how it feels to appreciate all that you have achieved in the last 30 days. Give thanks to everyone that has helped you along the way to achieve your goals. Do something extra special today that makes you really happy and see how that feels.

time to **reassess**

To allow more fun to enter your life, you must start with the belief that you really deserve to have enjoyment and relaxation in your life. Did you do everything you could this month to let go of old ideas that got in the way of having fun in either your personal or professional life?

Look at the funny side

There is a funny and serious side to all situations. When you get stuck in the mode of looking at everything from a serious point of view, even the simplest of decisions seems to take on monumental proportions. Allowing a bit of levity to enter the situation, lightens the load and removes any elements of jeopardy. Whenever you must make a big decision in life, think about the advice your favourite comedian might give you.

Have a good laugh

Laughter is a great way to dispel negative energy from your physical body, but, most importantly, it is quite contagious. Remember the universal truth of 'like attracts like' and laugh out loud more often. It is far more fun being around people who know how to appreciate a joke and enjoy life to the fullest. How has laughter improved your life in the last thirty days?

Nuture your relationships

Close family relations, friendships and love affairs thrive on attention. You need to acknowledge the special place that your friends occupy in your heart. Each of us craves recognition and appreciation for our special qualities, which we share with our most treasured of friends. Have you been feeling special because of a relation's, friend's or lover's thoughtful words or deeds? Have you learned what makes their soul sing?

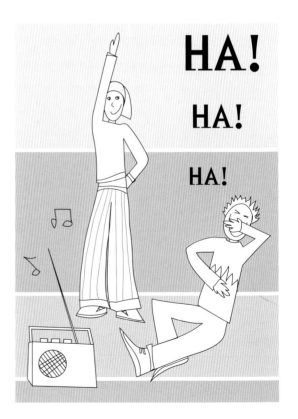

Benefit from relaxation

Incorporating relaxation strategies into your routine each and every day allows you to reap the physical benefits of giving your body and mind a much-needed rest. Have you felt the advantages of maintaining this discipline over the last thirty days? Are you able to concentrate more? Do you have more physical stamina?

Choose to have fun at work

Avoid the common trap of getting involved in office politics and gossip. Seek the ultimate satisfaction from your job, rather than just earning a living. Decide what you want from each segment of your day, put your heart and soul into it, and always choose the route that will be most fun. Fun stimulates the imagination and inflames passion. Live you life by the maxim that time flies when you are having fun.

Life is funnier than you thought

When you are having fun, you are receptive to new ideas and ways of interacting with those around you. By taking a conscious decision to look at ways of making each and every task you do a more enjoyable experience, you will alleviate much of the tension and pressure that you place yourself under, both in your personal and professional life.

When you find it difficult to laugh at the hand that life has dealt you, you stagnate and remain bogged down by the reality of what is. You hold on to negative emotions, such as anger, jealousy, and sadness, which physically prevent your body from relaxing and operating at peak levels. Simply by injecting a bit of lightness and humour into a situation, you are able to learn from your past mistakes, without it defeating your ego.

We are all modern day alchemists, with the ability to create magical moments for ourselves and for those who are important to us. By allowing others inside to share your innermost feelings, you gain acceptance and appreciation for who you truly are. By looking for the innermost feelings of others, you are able to enjoy more meaningful and intimate relationships. Have you found more enjoyment in your personal and professional life in the last thirty days as a result of seeking more fun out of life?

Make a new resolution

Go back and retake the Assess Your Relaxation Levels and Assess Your Fun Factor sections of the Postive Behaviour Survey on pages 28–31. See how your attitudes have changed in your personal and professional relationships. Are you more intimate with your partner and closer to your friends? Are you happier as a result? Are you spending more time doing the things you want to do, rather than those you feel you must do?

Now review the goals that you set for yourself from the Have Fun 30-day Action Plan. For each goal, answer the following questions. Do you feel more appreciated and loved as a result of looking at ways to appreciate and love your partner? Have you found that you get back what you give? Have you let go of old emotions that made you feel tense surrounding a member of your family? Are you able to look at the areas of similarity rather than contention? Have you developed stronger bonds with those you work with? Do you look for more ways of working together rather than separately? Are you able to turn humdrum tasks into personal competitions? Have you maintained your schedule of personal time?

Having fun is a conscious decision that you must take each time you start something new in your day, whether it is a daily chore, a new career or a burgeoning relationship. Remember, it takes just six weeks to form a habit. Keep going.

keep it going

It would be great if you could wave a magic wand and in a single instant have all that you desired. Or, would it? Having everything you ever wanted would leave little room for all the new and exciting experiences that come with desire and yearning. Each and every experience that you have in life is an important one. Without seeing the contrasts that life offers, it would be difficult to know what you really want. If every day were sunny, how would you know how refreshing the rain feels after a very humid day? Life requires contrasts to allow you to find your way.

In this age of technology, we now expect instant gratification. We want things to happen overnight, as if by magic. With many of the issues that you must face in life, there are years worth of beliefs, attitudes and emotions that you have attached to these issues, which may take time to work through and release. Each step that you take to resolve one of these issues, will release you from your past and allow you to feel the difference it makes to your emotions, mental attitude and physical presence.

We all go through life's ups and downs as a matter of course. How much you learn from each experience will dictate how many more times you will repeat them. Learning to accept that you are unable to change some situations in life will make the game more enjoyable. Expending energy on trying to change people and situations that you cannot control, only leads to frustration and resentment. One of the most important lessons to learn is that you are only able to control your own destiny by the decisions you take each and every day about yourself.

When you have some down time, it is important to learn from the experience. Keeping negative emotion buried inside simply means more work that will need to be done at a later time. Let out these feelings by using some of the emotional release techniques found throughout each chapter of this book and get on with life. You are only human, so you will sometimes lose your way. You must learn to always forgive others and yourself for any situation to get resolved.

Positive thinking is a choice you make over what feels better. In all instances, looking for the positive aspects of each situation makes you feel better about everything you do. If you practice looking at what you want from each situation, you will, over time, come to expect that you will get what you want. It takes a conscious effort for it to become a way of life. Always remember that it takes six weeks of constantly doing something in the same way for it to become a habit. Each time you lapse into old ways of thinking, you must consciously start the process over again.

Life is a game. How much fun you have, and what rewards you reap at the end of it, is totally dependent on how you play. Give it your best effort every step of the way and you will sort your life, achieve your dreams and have fun in the process.

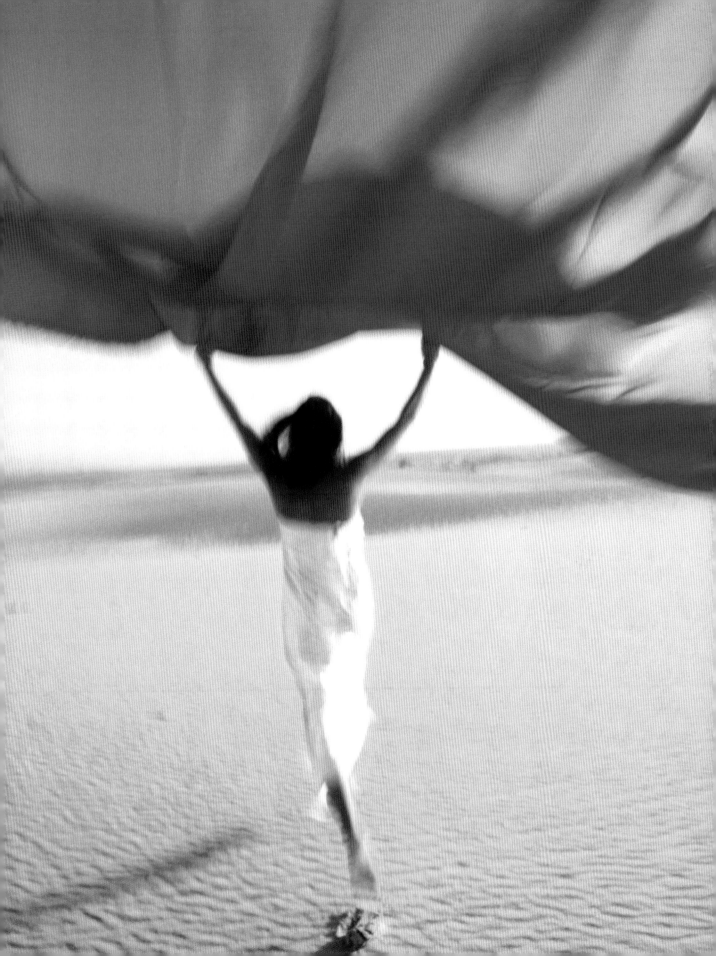

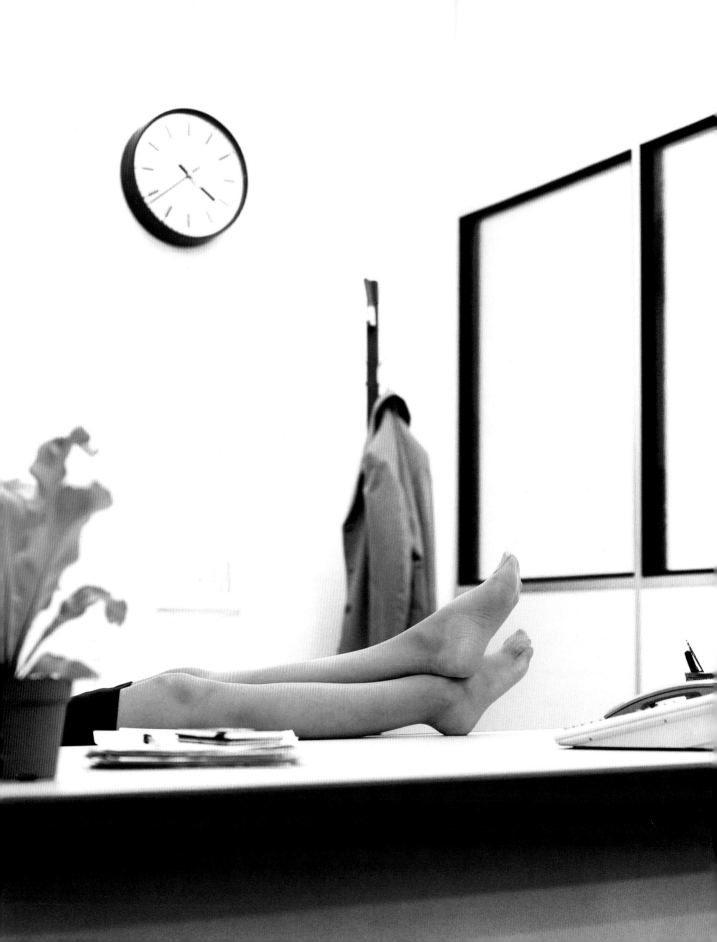

stay connected

To keep up the momentum and continue moving in a positive direction, it is necessary to take time out to observe where you are in the present moment. After the initial enthusiasm of getting going, you can begin to lapse slowly into bad habits and let areas of your life slip back to where they were.

You must always make a conscious effort to step back and view each situation in an observer's role to enable you to let go of the defence mechanisms that prohibit growth.

Make a date with yourself on a weekly basis and spend several hours observing where you are in the present moment. Do not look for the reasons why things are the way they are, just look at the way they are. From this vantage point you can move forward again to change those areas that are not as you wish them to be.

Imagine that you are a news writer or broadcaster sending back a dispatch from the frontline of your own life. As a journalist, you are following yourself around for an entire day, observing your physical, mental and emotional states as well as the physical environments that you inhabited.

Report only on what you observed about your general day-to-day situation, answering the following questions without adding any editorial comment. Remember to be entirely non-judgemental.

Do you feel healthy?

Are you eating a balanced diet?

Are you engaged in physical activities?

Do you spend time doing relaxing things?

Is your home neat with everything put away?

Is your office organised?

Are you spending time doing things you enjoy with friends and family?

Are you having fun in each activity?

Are you getting on with those around you?

Are you happy?

Review your answers and compare them to where you were when you first began reading in this book. Look for those areas that you have conquered and give yourself a pat on the back for continuing to progress on this positive path towards getting what you want. In those areas where you seem to have taken a step backwards, re-affirm your intention to improve the situation and use your creative tools of imagination and visualisation to envisage ways of changing the outcome.

Keeping it going takes a constant commitment to want to feel, look and be the best you can be. Re-direct your energy into giving each area you wish to change your undivided attention and enthusiasm. Do not take your eye off the ball.

keep editing

Leading a balanced life is a continual process of assessing what feels good to you in each and every moment. As you continue on the path towards achieving your dreams, it is necessary to let go of things that no longer serve a useful purpose or have ceased to bring you pleasure. Often this can be a difficult lesson to learn: it raises many emotional attachments you have to people, things and situations that, at one time, may have possessed a great deal of meaning in your life.

Learn to let go of the past. You need to understand that not all of the decisions you take in life lead you to what we really want. What you dream about today, most often bares no resemblance to what you dared to dream of even months ago. The important thing to keep in mind is that you change continually and, as a result, your tastes, attitudes and aspirations also change. Letting go of your old ways of thinking takes practice, but it makes room for new ideas.

Maintain the constant process of editing. Getting rid of any objects that you no longer use, which only take up valuable space in your home or office, produces particularly obvious benefits. By letting go of your unwanted items, you can enjoy more free space and the emotional benefits of a home that is not encumbered by the weight of the past. You are better positioned to appreciate the things you use, enjoy and treasure in the present, as they are easier to access. It also enables you to let go of the person you may have been when you first acquired those possessions and acknowledge who you are in the moment.

Acknowledge your past mistakes, learn from the experience and forgive yourself for your failings. All too often, we feel guilty about the choices we have made if they have been proven unsuccessful. You can feel reluctant to let go of things, especially when you have invested either money or time and effort in the process. Keeping the physical reminders, however, keeps you stuck in the past. It is essential to forgive yourself for being human and making mistakes in order to keep travelling forward on the right path in the present.

Lighten the load. There is no time like the present to make a clean sweep. Are there people, situations or material possessions in your life that you still need to let go? For each thing you shed, you will create space for a new experience or item to take its place.

List all the things that you have outgrown in your current circumstances. Start with the easiest item first – something with the least emotional attachment – and take action today to clear it away. Once you have experienced how good it feels to let go of something that no longer serves a purpose and have enjoyed the associated benefits, progress on to the more

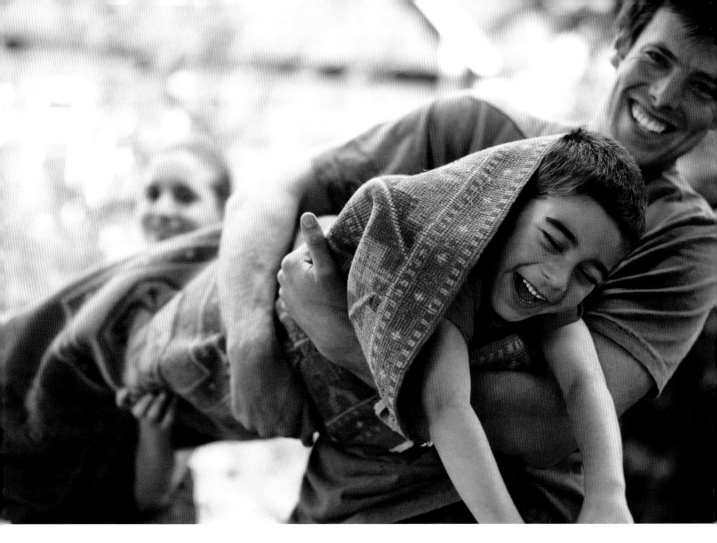

emotionally loaded objects. Set aside one day
of uninterrupted time to go through your
possessions and edit them down to the essentials
– either things that you use or things that you
love and make you happy.

Release any negative emotions that are
holding you back. Re-assess any past situations or
emotions that are preventing you from achieving
your dreams. Go back to the Open Your Heart
Positive Action Exercise on pages 106–7 to
release these negative emotions. If you find that
you are involved in relationships that no longer
bring you joy, what are you waiting for? Make the
break and let only those people who make you
feel good about yourself into your life. You are the
only one responsible for the rest of your life.

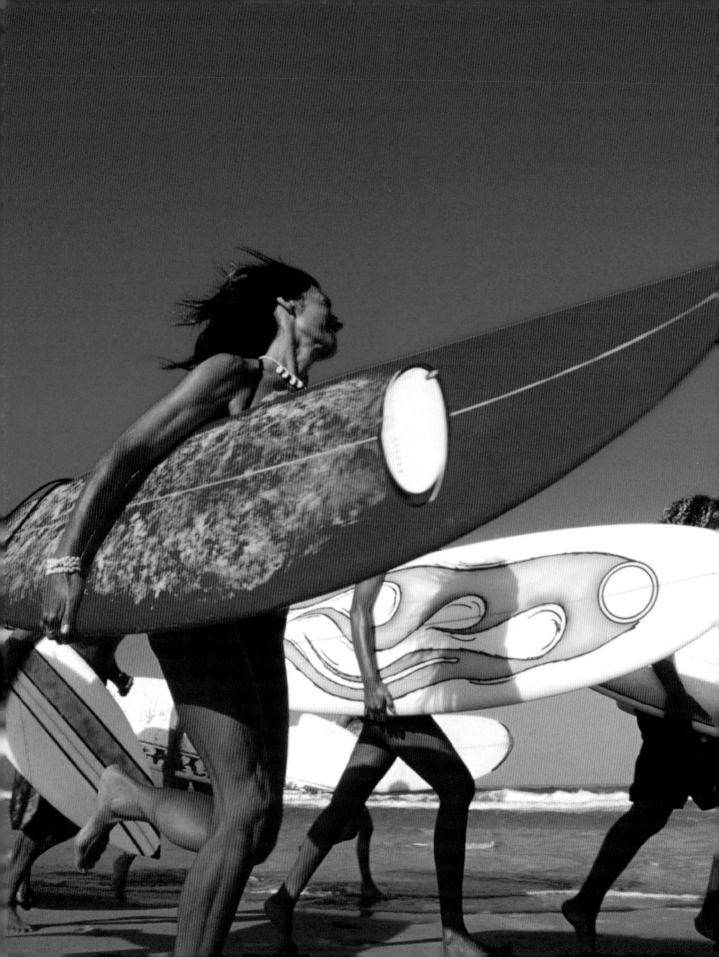

take a fresh approach

Whenever life becomes too routine, you tend to switch off and go through the motions. If the outcome is predictable, your expectations will be limited. You simply stop putting in the effort and find that things start to stagnate. You get stale, just like a body of water that does not flow.

Never fear the unknown. Going for it means that you are willing to be all that you can be, not just what you are at the moment. You will only be able to reach this state of being by releasing your fears of the unknown and giving things a go. You need stimulation, each and every day, to provide the added excitement of the limitless possibilities that lie around the next bend.

Learn something new each day. There are no failures in life, only lessons to be learned. Without learning new tricks, Jack becomes a dull boy. By setting your intention to have a new experience you will be open to them when they present themselves. Most often it is as a result of letting other people into your life who can help you on your path of development, and listening to what they have to say. Each new thing you learn adds to your cumulative experience and changes the way you view the world.

Kick-start change in your life. Take a look at the areas of your life that could still use a bit of stimulation. When you look at them closely, you will probably find that you are continuing to focus on what you do not like about the situation, rather than all that it brings to your life. By giving it a kick-start with fresh, new ideas, you will find the joy in the situation becomes easier to obtain.

Make a list of routine tasks that you undertake on a daily basis, and position them in order of how much you enjoy doing them, starting with those that you least enjoy doing.

Getting ready for the day

Going to work

Doing household chores

Spending time with family or friends

Going to bed

For each task, think of five new ways of doing it. Consider changing the time or location that you normally undertake these actions, or bringing new people into the situation to get a different point of view. Think of changing the physical space around you, or of taking new methods of transportation to give you added stimulus. Think about going to new places. Think about changing colours or adding fragrances to uplift your spirit. Most of all, simply think about the endless ways there are to make the experience more fun. Now go out and try each and every thing you have thought about to liven up the situation. See all the possibilities that this wonderful universe has in store.

appreciate your achievements

The more you are able to acknowledge your innate abilities, the more comfortable you will be in trusting your inner guidance system to help you achieve all that you are capable of. Keeping your personal progress moving forward in the right direction requires that you take the time to appreciate your efforts, regardless of how great or small you feel they may be. Spend a moment each day evaluating how far you have come; you will soon see the results of your actions.

How do you feel about what is going on in your life right now? Are you taking 100 percent responsibility for all your actions? Do you look for the positive aspects of each situation and everything that you learned as a result?

You need to understand that for every action you take, there is a reaction. Life is a continual cycle of cause and effect. Your current circumstances are a result of everything you have done in the past. Considering your daily actions will help you to see more clearly how the choices you make impact on what you have created.

Each and everything you do has a purpose and a lesson to be learned from the experience. Whether you succeed or fail is often irrelevant. Rather than the achievement, it is the learning of the lesson that helps the growth process, and allows you to blossom.

I find this quote from Ralph Waldo Emerson particularly inspiring, 'What lies behind us and what lies before us are tiny matters, compared to what lies within us.' I hope you do too.

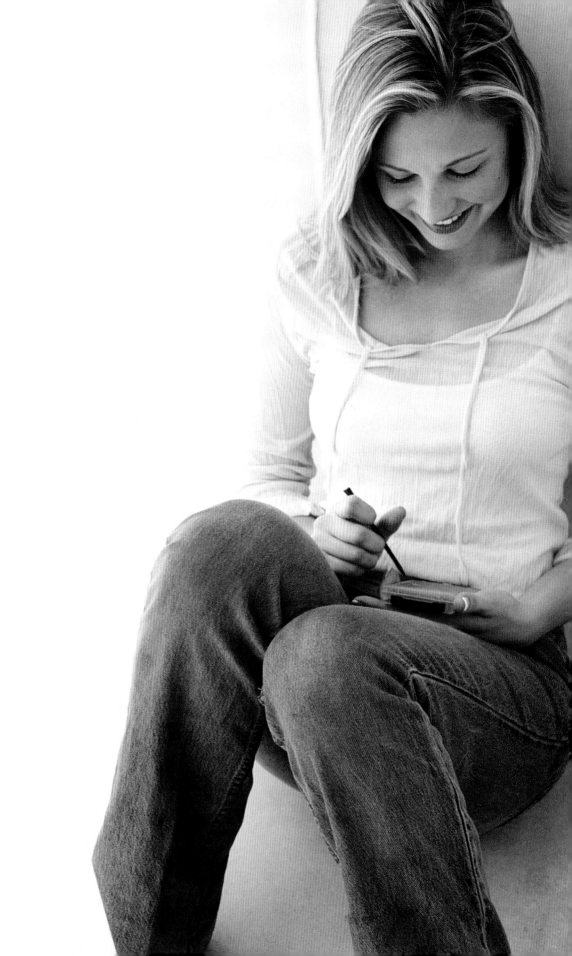

further information

Further reading

Organisation and de-cluttering

The Life Laundry
by Dawna Walter and Mark Franks,
BBC Worldwide, 2002.

New Leaf, New Life by Dawna Walter,
Quadrille Publishing, 2001

Organized Living
by Dawna Walter with Helen Chislett,
Conran Publishing, 1999

Clear Your Clutter with Feng Shui
by Karen Kingston, Piatkus, 1998

Calm at Work by Paul Wilson,
Penguin Books, 1998

Healing Methods

Reiki and The Healing Buddha
by Maureen Kelly,
Full Circle, 2001 (Indian edition)

The Healing Handbook by Tara Ward,
Arcturus, 2000

Miracles of Mind
by Russell Targ and Jane Katra Ph.D.,
New World Library, 1998

Vibrational Medicine by Richard Gerber, M.D.,
Bear & Company, 2001

Essential Reiki by Diane Stein,
The Crossing Press Inc.,1995

Spiritual Development

Anatomy of the Spirit by Caroline Myss, Ph.D,
Bantam, 1999

Soul Mates by Thomas Moore,
Element Books Ltd., 1994

A Harmony of Angels by Angela McGerr,
Quadrille Publishing, 2001

A Path with Heart by Jack Kornfield,
Bantam, 1993

The Artist's Way by Julia Cameron,
Souvenir Press, 1994

For further development

Helplines:

Bereavement
Cruse Bereavement Line
tel 0870 167 1677
www.caritas.data.co.uk

Emotional Support
Samaritans
tel 0845 790 9090
www.samaritans.org.uk

Daily Motivation

Thought for Today
www.innerspace.org.uk/
home/thoughtfortoday.asp

Self Development

Free courses on self development
www.brahmakumaris.org.uk

Aromatherapy
International Federation of Aromatherapists
tel 020 8742 2605
www.int-fed-aromatherapy.co.uk

Crystal Healing
Affiliation of Crystal Healing Organisations
tel 020 8398 7252

Feng Shui
Feng Shui Network International
tel 070 0033 6474
www.fengshuinet.com

Homeopathy
Society of Homeopaths
tel 01604 621400
www.homeopathy-soh.org

Meditation
Transcendental Meditation
tel 0800 269303

Reiki
Dr Allan J. Sweeney
International Reiki Healing and Training Centre
www.reiki-healing.com

The Science of Deliberate Creation
www.abraham-hicks.com

Spiritual Healing
National Federation of Spiritual Healers
tel 0891 616 080

Stress Management
International Stress
Management Organisation
www.isma.org.uk

T'ai Chi
T'ai Chi Association UK
tel 020 7407 4775
www.taichiuk.co.uk

Yoga
British Wheel of Yoga
tel 01529 306851
www.bwy.org.uk

Home and office organisation

Aero tel 020 7351 0511

Bureau tel 020 7379 7898

The Conran Shop tel 020 75897401
www.conran.co.uk

Habitat tel 020 7631 3880
www.habitat.net

Harrods tel 020 7235 5000

Heals tel 020 7636 1666

The Holding Company tel 020 7352 1600
www.theholdingcompany.co.uk

Homebase tel 020 8749 6982

Ikea UK Ltd tel 020 8208 5600

Jerry's Home Store tel 020 7581 0909

John Lewis Partnership tel 020 7629 7711

Liberty tel 020 7734 1234

Muji tel 020 7352 7148

Next tel 0845 600 7000

Ocean tel 020 7670 1234

index

acknowledgments

Author's acknowledgments

Dedicated to the angel in all of us.

With special thanks to Jane, Lisa, Helen, Jim and Coralie at Quadrille Publishing. My husband, Jerry, for always being a cheerleader and having enormous faith in my abilities. My mother Gooch and sisters for encouraging me from childhood to be all that I could be. Allan Sweeney for his inspired teaching and healing methods. Al, Annie, Bhimi, Caroline, Cat, Celia, Christopher, David, Debs, Delacy, Elias, Ellen, Emma, Gillie, Grant, Jane, John, Judy, Karen, Kate, Kerry, Linda, Lynda, Nina, Matt, Matthew, Mike, Mohini, Nicola, Pattie, Phil, Rupert, Ruth, Sally, Sam, Sarah, Sarina, Sergio, Susie, Tessa, Tibye, Tom, Victor and all of my other inspiring friends who always bring me joy. The fur children – Sydney, Lola, Angel, Cosmo and Figgy – for their intuitive healing powers. All my friends at The Life Laundry who make things happen every day.

Publisher's acknowledgments

1 and 104 Robert Harding/Sydney Shaffer; 2 Gettyimages/Stephen Simpson; 9 Gettyimages/Frederic Lucano; 11 ImageState; 12 Camera Press/*Brigitte*; 15 Taverne Agency/Hotze Eisma/Hanne Lise Poli; 19 ImageState; 35 Camera Press; 36 ImageState; 39 Gettyimages/Justin Pumfrey; 40 Photonica/Neo Vision; 43 Camera Press; 47 IPC Syndication/© *Living Etc.*/Sandra Lane; 48 Gettyimages/David Roth; 53 IPC Syndication/© *Living Etc.*/Chris Everard; 54 Gettyimages/Ken Reid; 57 ImageState; 60 ImageState; 67 Gettyimages/Tobi Corney; 68 Gettyimages/V.C.L.; 71 Gettyimages/Alexander Walter; 72 Gettyimages/Victoria Pearson; 77 Gettyimages/Brian Bailey; 78 ImageState; 81 Camera Press/Vital; 82 Gettyimages/PS Productions; 87 ImageState; 88 Gettyimages/Barry Yee; 99 Gettyimages/Jean Louis Batt; 100 IPC Syndication/© Me Magazine; 103 Gettyimages/Stephanie Rausser; 109 Gettyimages/Vcl/Spencer Rowell; 110 Gettyimages/Mark Douet; 113 Gettyimages/Steve Taylor; 117 Gettyimages/Adri Berger; 118 IPC Syndication/© Living Etc./David Clerihew; 121 Gettyimages/Jean-Marc Scialom; 124 Robert Harding/Michelangelo Gratton; 131 ImageState; 132 Gettyimages/Kelvin Murray; 135 ImageState; 136 Gettyimages/Mark Douet; 139 Gettyimages/Steven Lam.